In our chemically ladened world, we must educate ourselves and find ways to improve our own health. Dr. Behzad Azargoshasb, ND, in his book, *Rules of Health*, makes this an easy transition for us. His book provides you with the knowledge to easily incorporate a holistic approach in your day to day living, so that you can make healthy living part of your lifestyle by introducing small habits that are easily sustainable. If you are looking to change the path your health is on, I highly recommend *Rules of Health*.

—Jacquie Lombardi, CEO of Kaizen Health Group, Mississauga, Ontario

Rules of Health is a book I would recommend to all my patients. If you implement these simple yet powerful rules, a healthier life is assured. Moreover, this book can be your regular reference for different stages of life. Simply put, *Rules of Health* is as close to a "magic pill" as you can get.

—Dr. Saisi Yang, ND, Vitality Physical Medicine

Dr. Behzad is a master at laying the groundwork for everyone who wants to get their health back on track. I would wish for all of my patients to read this practical resource before coming to see me—it would make my work a whole lot easier!

—Dr. Freda Tam, ND, VIDA Massage & Wellness and
Balanced Living Massage Therapy & Wellness Centre

Rules of Health is such an effortless read and so elegantly describes the fundamentals for a healthy and happy life. Not only are each of these factors more relevant than ever in everyday life, but the words offer so much insight and usefulness for everyone. This book serves as one of the most authentic and comprehensive resources for healthy living.

—Rishi Mehta, naturopathic student

This book gives simple and effective advice on how to lead a healthy life. I like how it is categorized in air, water, food, sleep, exercise, stress, relationships, detox, cancer prevention, weight management, pregnancy, kids, mental health and aging. All of these areas will affect one's wellbeing, and knowing the strategies to optimize each category is extremely empowering. Dr. Azargoshasb ties in all of the basic principles for a healthy life in an elegant package. A must-read for anyone who wants a guide to optimize their health without the overwhelming medical jargon.

—Dr. Cecilia de Martino, ND, Willow Wellness Clinic

RULES
of
Health

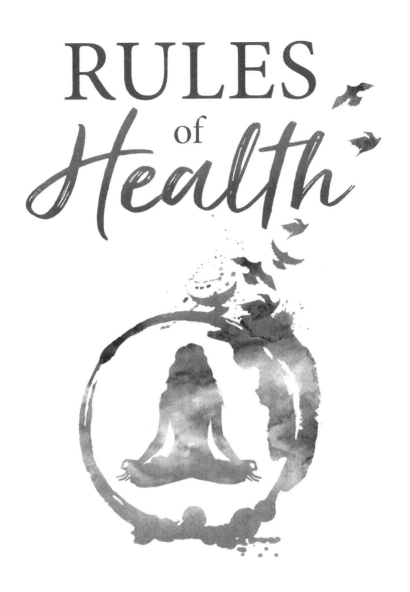

Behzad Azargoshasb

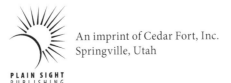

An imprint of Cedar Fort, Inc.
Springville, Utah

I dedicate this book to you, my reader.
May it inspire and motivate you onto a healthier lifestyle.

ISBN 13: 978-1-4621-2272-1

Published by Plain Sight Publishing, an imprint of Cedar Fort, Inc.
2373 W. 700 S., Springville, UT 84663
Distributed by Cedar Fort, Inc., www.cedarfort.com

LIBRARY OF CONGRESS CATALOGING-IN-PUBLICATION DATA

Names: Azargoshasb, Behzad, 1979- author.
Title: Rules of health : sustaining optimal health through safe
   detoxification, reaching a healthy weight, managing stress effectively,
   and achieving deep restorative sleep / Behzad Azargoshasb.
Description: Springville, Utah : Plain Sight Publishing, an imprint of Cedar
   Fort, Inc., [2018] | Includes bibliographical references and index.
Identifiers: LCCN 2018027877 (print) | LCCN 2018029848 (ebook) | ISBN
   9781462129478 (epub, pdf, mobi) | ISBN 9781462122721 (perfect bound : alk.
   paper)
Subjects: LCSH: Health--Popular works.
Classification: LCC RA776 (ebook) | LCC RA776 .A93 2018 (print) | DDC
   613--dc23
LC record available at https://lccn.loc.gov/2018027877

Cover design by Shawnda T. Craig
Cover design © 2018 Cedar Fort, Inc.
Edited by Valene Wood and James Gallagher (Castle Walls Editing LLC)
Typeset by Kaitlin Barwick

Printed in the United States of America

10 9 8 7 6 5 4 3 2 1

Printed on acid-free paper

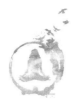

Contents

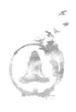

Introduction

A s a naturopathic doctor, my main objective when treating patients is to help them achieve their optimal health by finding and treating the root cause of their health concern. Going one step further, the philosophy of "prevention is the best medicine" is what I promote with all my patients, who unfortunately are trapped in a sick care system that places little value on preventative health measures. Don't get me wrong. There is a time and place for all types of medical interventions, and they do provide a valuable service, when needed.

I believe that you are a smart consumer of health information, which is what attracted you to this book. As a health-savvy individual, you may have realized that true health is best achieved through healthy living habits. We are integrated beings. Every part of our being is connected with every other part. An imbalance in one part will create an imbalance in other locations. This loss in equilibrium can manifest itself both internally within our bodies and externally in our environment. Therefore, we cannot treat the problem at the surface level and expect it to go away. Until all the interconnected organ systems and environmental factors are balanced, the health issue will persist.

For example, heart disease is not just a disease of the heart. It influences other organ systems and, to a certain level, is influenced by one's psychological well-being. The underlying cause for heart disease may have been long-term stress that increased stress hormones, leading to high blood sugar. High blood sugar will trigger insulin production to lower it, and being consistently stressed may lead to low blood sugar levels (hypoglycemia), among other consequences. To overcome hypoglycemia, people crave and consume ready-made comfort foods on a regular basis, and these are usually loaded with sugar, fat, and a cocktail of unhealthy ingredients. This habit may lead to unsafe visceral fat deposits within the abdominal cavity, putting pressure on organs such as the liver, pancreas, and kidneys, while disrupting hormone regulation. Over time, high psychological stress levels desensitize people to the regulatory effects of stress hormones on inflammation within the body, and this starts an inflammatory process that affects susceptible organ systems.[1] Furthermore, because of stress, one may become more sedentary, lack motivation to exercise, and start smoking to relieve anxiety. Smoking, along with visceral fat, has raised the possibility of blockages forming in the arteries supplying blood to the heart muscles. In cases like this, it is only a matter of time before a heart attack occurs.

Does this sound familiar? As you can see, it isn't a single reason that leads to an individual's health demise but a cascade of events slowly doing hidden damage until the body shouts out for attention. In such cases, what do you think is the correct course of action? One could address the smoking issue or advocate consuming less unhealthy food or recommend taking medication to overcome the detrimental effects of these behaviors, and these actions would all help, to a certain extent. However, if you said that the individual first needs to reduce or manage stress levels, you are on the right path. If we are to ever restore health, we must try to get at the root cause of the issue and address it in a holistic way.

There is no such thing as perfect health, and if someone tries to sell you on a formula or recipe for perfect health, turn and run. Optimum health lies on a continuum. It is an ever-evolving and dynamic process within you. You will have good days when you feel amazing, physically and emotionally, and you will have bad days when you want to curl up in bed and disappear. But most of the time you will have normal days. That is real life. All you can do as a human being is try to achieve your individual best health, which may be different from someone else's. If you are on the cusp of healthiness, which is the case for many folks, then you are not alone. It takes time to acquire good health, and it takes effort to stay healthy. My goal is to make it easier for you in your healing journey, so you will have many more days when you feel incredible and are able to overcome health challenges that come your way.

Imagine that you own a car that you drive twenty-four hours a day. This car is a special-edition, handmade machine, and no other like it has ever been made. Another great thing about this car is that if you maintain it well, which you have, it will last a good eighty to one hundred years. You have never had to replace any tires or brakes, and it still has the original engine and transmission. Any time you had scratches or dents, your car would magically heal itself. All you had to give it was high-quality fuel and regular oil changes, nothing else. You made sure you didn't drive it rough and it always had one driver: you.

But when you look at your neighbor's car, it's a different story. He was not so fortunate. He was rough with his car right from the beginning; it had multiple drivers, all of whom abused the car. He would forget to change the oil and run the engine almost dry. He would speed and brake hard. He never put in the right fuel. He had to replace many components, costing him a fortune. Over the years, his car has gotten into really bad shape and looks like it won't survive much longer.

As you may have already deduced, the car is an analogy for your body. I would suggest that you read the paragraph again and try to appreciate the deeper meaning. We all have a remarkable and miraculous self-healing machine, and all it requires is some tender loving care to stay strong and healthy and give you years of good service and pleasure. What more can one ask for? I offer this analogy to emphasize the importance of healthy lifestyle habits for achieving good health. Most chronic diseases take years of unhealthy behaviors to develop, and it's usually simple, routine things we do unknowingly that cause damage. Just like the car, your body needs wholesome food and regular upkeep to stay healthy. This includes essentials like sufficient exercise, stress management, and quality sleep. It sounds easy enough, but in our present world, it can be a challenge to do these basic things with consistency.

This is where the "Rules of Health" come into play. I have broken down healthy living into its fundamentals: simple things that, if done with consistency, will provide amazing health benefits. There are no gimmicks and no programs to follow. This book aims to be your ultimate guide to healthy living. Most of what is discussed forms the foundation of how to live a healthy life physically, mentally, and emotionally. I would normally discuss these topics with my patients during several visits. When my patients start to follow these simple suggestions, they see a profound improvement in their health, with less need for medical intervention. My intention is to inform and inspire you so that you can incorporate most of the suggestions into your own life as best you can and watch the magic happen. I hope you enjoy the book and find it of value in your life.

In good health,
yours sincerely,
Dr. Behzad Azargoshasb, ND
Naturopathic doctor, author
www.facebook.com/docwriterunleashed

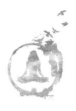

RULES FOR *Air*

When one thinks about breathing, an immediate association with life comes to mind, as in the "Breath of Life." For those of us who have no difficulty breathing, it happens seamlessly and effortlessly, but ask someone with lung disease and you will know how precious breathing is. As you may remember from science class, one of the main functions of breathing is to allow the absorption of oxygen and the release of carbon dioxide. Our bodies maintain a delicate balance of these two molecules in the blood, and without this balance we would literally die within a matter of minutes. Hence, I start this book with the most important thing you can do for your health.

1: Breathe Slowly, Breathe Deeply

Our cells need oxygen to produce energy. If you sometimes feel like you lack energy even though you slept great and are well rested, your breathing may be the issue. Most people are chest breathers. You may ask, how else are we supposed to breathe? We should be breathing using our diaphragm, the strong dome-shaped muscle under our lungs primarily responsible for breathing. This process of breathing will be explained in detail shortly. If you are a chest breather, you will notice two things. One is that your chest will rise and fall with every inhalation and exhalation. Second, your breathing will be more frequent. This form of breathing will only fill your lungs partially with air and not use the full capacity of your lungs for oxygen absorption.

2: When to Go See a Doctor

Breathing should always be natural and never forced. If you have to consistently use extra energy to breathe or if you start developing shortness of breath without physical exertion, then it's a possible medical issue, and you should let your doctor know. This rule only applies when you don't have a cold or the flu, during which time your nasal passages can get congested and you may be compelled to breathe through your mouth.

3: Inside Air v. Outside Air

The air in our homes can get a lot dirtier than outside air because of how air-tight modern homes can be. And since we spend so much time in our homes, it would only make sense to ensure that the air we are breathing is clean and free of toxins. If you have a forced-air heating and cooling system, use a HEPA (high-efficiency particulate air) filter and change the filter every season or, depending on how thick the filter is, at least once a year. This will ensure you are breathing clean and purified air, free of pollutants, and it will extend the life of your furnace as well. If you don't have a central-air circulation system, like in an apartment, then there are portable air purifiers available at different sizes and prices. As before, make sure it uses a high-quality filter and at least have one in your bedroom. We sleep, on average, a third of our lives; let's make sure we breathe clean air during that time. In the spring and autumn months, when the outside air hovers between 10°C and 20°C (or between 50°F and 68°F), the home's heating and cooling system doesn't work as much, and hence the air in the house can get even more polluted. Make sure to open the windows during these months. Opening windows on the opposite ends of the house is more effective at creating a cross circulation of fresh air. The goal is to minimize breathing in polluted air in the place where you spend most of your time.

4: What to Do about Those Dreaded Allergies

If you suffer from seasonal allergies, my heart goes out to you. The most common symptoms associated with these airborne allergies are clear, runny nose along with bouts of sneezing, itchy or teary eyes, and scratchy throat, sometimes with ear congestion and postnasal drainage, which can trigger a dry cough. A lot of people simply endure this nuisance, but there are simple approaches you can take to avoid being hit by the worst.

To begin with, if you are not already doing so, resist going outside during a high pollen count. If you have allergies to pollen from specific trees or grass, then a smart option would be to use a weather app that informs you of their daily levels. Factors that can change the pollen count in the air include wind speed, temperature, humidity, and the species of grass and trees in the area (as well as where along in the season they are). Pollen count can change day to day, but early-season grass pollen counts tend to peak twice during the day, once around mid-morning and again in the evening. By late season, the pollen counts tend to peak once around midday.[1] This pattern is seen in European studies. The pattern may change slightly, depending on where you live. Plan your activities to avoid being outdoors during those peaks.

If you suffer from allergies throughout the year and your home is carpeted, vacuum it regularly. Animals can catch pollen on their fur when outdoors, so have someone vacuum them right away if they have been out for a while. Also consider using a HEPA air purifier in the room where you spend most of your time. It can be effective at alleviating the symptoms associated with your airborne allergies. Individuals with seasonal allergies generally have an immune dysfunction that causes their immune system to get hypersensitive to seemingly harmless airborne particles.

If seasonal allergies are making your life miserable, then it may be helpful to visit an expert. The most common way to treat the symptoms is to take antihistamine medication. If you would like to go the natural route, you can modulate the immune system with specific nutrients and botanicals, something a naturopathic doctor would be trained in.

5: Are You Spending Too Much Time in Your Car?

In the United States, most people spend on average a little less than an hour each day commuting to and from work.[2] Some people can attest to spending much more time than that in their cars. The time spent commuting can start to creep up if you live in a congested city. The air in our cars can also get toxic from fumes released by the car interior and gases that seep through. As a general rule, as soon as you get in the car, put the windows down for a short while to bring in fresh air. Also try to replace the cabin air filter of your car regularly, at least once every two years, more often if you live in a dusty or polluted place.

6: Simple Ways to Keep the Air Clean

Clean air is a luxury few of us have. Try your best not to contribute to air pollution, and maximize the ways you can improve the air quality in your environment. The following are some of the best ways to do that:

- Stop smoking. If you are a smoker, then consider quitting for good.
- Drive greener cars. If you don't have a fuel-efficient car, keeping your car well maintained may help to reduce its toxic emissions.
- Don't barbecue with charcoal often; barbecue with gas instead.
- Don't use a lot of products with propellant sprays, like aerosol air fresheners, hair products, or cleaning products. Get the equivalent product in a non-spray version. The propellants used in these products may be toxic. If they are used in an enclosed space, you or your loved ones could breathe them in.
- Don't support companies and organizations that are not concerned with their environmental impact. Instead, support those that care about what we leave behind for our children. The best way to bring about change is with your pocketbook. By purchasing products and

services from green companies, you are, in effect, supporting and encouraging innovations and change for the better.

- Plant trees whenever you get a chance. If you have a big backyard without any trees, consider planting fruit-producing trees suited for the climate. You will get lots of free fruit, increase the value of your property, and help the environment as well. If you don't have land to grow trees, most municipalities have tree-planting programs that take volunteers to parks and other conservation areas to plant different species of trees. Growing trees in an urban environment can sequester large amounts of carbon dioxide and pollutants and clean the air, which can have a significant impact on air quality and human health.[3]

- Get indoor plants to beautify your home and to purify the indoor air. Most plants will do a good job at removing toxins from the air, but according to a NASA study, plants like peace lily, chrysanthemum, snake plant, English ivy, and bamboo palm seem to do a better job at removing toxins such as trichloroethylene, formaldehyde, benzene, xylene, and ammonia.[4]

- Another aspect of indoor air pollution that is often missed is off-gassing from new items in your home, such as furniture, electronics, bedding, and cleaning products. If you ever get a new car, the classic new-car smell is attributable to volatile organic compounds (VOCs) released by the car's interior upholstery. Try your best to purchase large items during the warmer months, when you can air out your home easily for a few weeks until the off-gassing has subsided. This will prevent the buildup of these toxic chemicals in your home and, ultimately, in your body. Do the same with your new car. Drive with the windows down for a couple of months until the new-car smell has diminished.

7: If You Live with a Smoker

To avoid secondhand smoke, which can be just as deadly to the people living in the house as it is to the smoker, make sure people never smoke in the house. Even in the bathroom with the exhaust on is not acceptable. If you have small kids, then they could also get exposed to thirdhand smoke from the smoker's clothes. Make sure the smoker does not handle a child after smoking. An even better solution is for them to have a separate set of clothes for smoking.

8: If You Are a Smoker

I am not going to try to convince you to quit smoking. This is a decision you have to make on your own. I am sure you are aware of the dangers associated with long-term exposure not only to you, but to everyone around you. If you are not aware, then I would suggest that you educate yourself. Spend time with people who have had complications from smoking, such as cancer, emphysema, or vascular difficulties. Hear their hardships and feel what it would be like to experience those things.

It's not easy to quit smoking. The nicotine in tobacco cigarettes is very addictive, and, as with any addiction, it feeds a need in you. It may improve your mood and performance and reduce anxiety levels, and with time it becomes second nature. Quitting smoking is not just letting go of one habit. It is letting go of several habits, such as when you smoke, where you smoke, what you smoke, how you smoke, and under what circumstances you must smoke. Since it's a habit-driven behavior, your highest success in quitting can be achieved by breaking the habit with other habits of a less-destructive nature. This needs to be done gradually, breaking and replacing each habit slowly.

Address the underlying reason you started smoking. If you are highly stressed, then adopt coping mechanisms such as deep breathing or meditation. Meditation seems to have a high success rate in improving self-control.[5] If you can, get the help of professionals who can guide you with their expertise. Keep yourself accountable to others and focus on the health benefits of quitting smoking. Use reasons such as staying alive for loved ones to keep you motivated. This won't be easy, but it's doable. Thousands of people have successfully quit smoking, and you can too. Good luck.

9: Laugh Frequently

Laughter is an exercise for the lungs and greatly increases oxygen intake. Laughter also reduces stress levels and improves natural killer-cell activity within our immune system.[6] To stimulate laughter, you can watch comedies frequently, go out with friends and laugh, or join a laughter yoga club. Think of laughter as medicine that keeps on giving to motivate you to find the funny in everyday situations and laugh to your heart's content.

10: Notice Your Breathing

Are you breathing fast or shallow? If you are, notice your emotions and the environment you are in. Most times we are unaware that when we get anxious, angry, or sad, our breathing cycle gets disrupted. When you do feel under the influence of a strong emotion, slow down your breathing and do the following:

- Slowly count in your head, breathing in to a count of three and breathing out to a count of five. Inhale and exhale only through your nose.
- Do this three times. Now notice your emotions again.

- Did you realize what triggered the original emotion in you? Start by being more aware of your surroundings and your emotional triggers.
- Most of the time, we cannot avoid the situations or individuals that upset us. If you are in such a position, then close your eyes and take three slow, deep breaths before confronting the individual or situation. This will allow you to lower your stress levels and put you in a headspace where you can calmly and rationally deal with it.

11: Breathe like a Baby

If you have ever noticed infants breathing, their bellies rise with every inhalation and fall on every exhalation. To breathe like this, lie down and put one hand on your belly, right on top of your belly button. Put the other one right in the middle of your chest. Now imagine that you have a balloon in your belly that you are trying to fill with air. As you breathe in, your belly should rise and your chest should stay mostly stationary. This happens as the lungs fill maximally and push the digestive organs away, giving them a nice massage in the process. As you breathe out, the belly will fall naturally because of gravity and tissue elasticity. You can also put a heavy book on your belly to assist you with this technique. Later on, after a few practice sessions, try this breathing technique while seated or standing with your back straight. Try to slow down your breath as much as you can without forcing yourself or becoming uncomfortable, always making sure your exhalation is slightly longer than your inhalation. This type of breathing is called belly breathing, more technically known as diaphragmatic breathing.

Breathe like this at least ten times every night before bed, and you will sleep like a baby. Whenever you are stressed, close your eyes and do three belly breaths, paying attention to the movement of your breath, and see how you feel. Initially, as you practice this type of breathing, placing the hands on the chest and belly helps to give you visual and tactile cues. But once you feel yourself belly breathing naturally, you don't need the hand placement. With time you will notice that your new breathing style will have you more energized and relaxed at the same time.

Another important thing to notice while breathing is your posture, specifically how hunched your back is. You may notice that as you slouch, it gets more difficult to take in a good breath. Make it a practice to observe and correct your posture regularly and see the effects in your life.

12: The Missing Piece of the Puzzle, "Humidity"

Another aspect of air that is frequently overlooked is the humidity. The amount of moisture in the air determines the humidity, and both high and low humidity can contribute to adverse health effects. If you live in a cold climate, then chances are that during the winter months indoor relative humidity may fall below 40 percent unless your home is humidified. Low humidity allows the flu virus to live longer and spread easier, as the nasal passages and sinuses can dry up, reducing your protection against these bugs. By increasing the humidity above 40 percent, we decrease the cases of respiratory infections as well as lessen the severity of asthmatic and allergic attacks.

Just as low humidity is a concern, high humidity above 60 percent, which occurs mostly in the summer months, comes with its own host of problems. Fungi, mold, and mites thrive in high-humidity environments. Furthermore, high humidity encourages rapid off-gassing of formaldehyde from furniture, plywood, carpets, and other structures whose relative concentration in the air is directly proportional to the relative humidity.[7]

I would recommend maintaining your home's humidity between 40 and 60 percent. During the winter months, using evaporative or steam humidifiers can help. During the summer months, you can use a dehumidifier. It would be prudent to do the same for your work environment by citing the importance of the correct level of humidity to your employer.

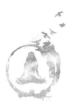

RULES FOR *Water*

It may not seem like it, but we are essentially walking containers of water. Over 60 percent of your body is composed of water.[1] Water is used within the body for many processes, and even a small drop in hydration levels can be noticeable. When you are dehydrated, you can feel your mind is not as sharp as usual. You may get headaches frequently, your energy levels are not what they normally are, and you get constipated more easily.

According to a study by the Centers for Disease Control and Prevention (CDC), 43 percent of adults drink less than four cups of water a day[2]; we are experiencing a dehydration epidemic. It would only seem logical that one of the biggest influences you can have over your health is to pay attention to your hydration level. Follow the instructions below to keep your water needs in check.

1: How to Know Your Water Requirements

Just as proper breathing is essential to health, drinking enough pure water is paramount to your well-being, so try to make it a priority in your life. There are two main indicators for adequate water consumption: thirst and the color of your urine. Your body will signal that you are getting dehydrated by the sensation of thirst. Don't ignore this sensation, and drink a glass of H_2O. According to an Australian study, when you have consumed enough water, you will feel resistance in your swallowing reflex and it will become physically more difficult to swallow.[3] So the lesson here is to listen to your body and you will be just fine.

When it comes to urine, if your urine is transparent to light yellow most of the time, then you are drinking enough water. If it is transparent all the time, then you are probably drinking more water than you need. That is nothing to worry about in most cases, as healthy kidneys can efficiently remove excess water and preserve blood electrolyte and mineral balance. That does not mean you can go overboard and drink excessive amounts of water, as water intoxication can be lethal. On the other end of the spectrum, if your urine is frequently darker yellow to orange, you may be dehydrated. It is better to be well hydrated than dehydrated any day of the week, especially if you are someone who struggles with fatigue and weight issues. Hydration is an important aspect in successful weight loss and management.

2: When to Go See a Doctor

If you are thirsty all the time outside of physical exertion or a hot climate, which is forcing you to drink lots of water and urinate constantly, then you may have a medical issue such as diabetes—get it checked out.

Certain foods and medications can change your urine color temporarily, but if your urine stays darker in spite of drinking adequate water, or if it suddenly changes color into the red or brown hues and stays that way consistently, then you could have kidney or liver issues—get it checked out.

3: Learn to Distinguish between Thirst and Hunger

The area of your brain that controls thirst and hunger is in a small region of the brain called the hypothalamus, which controls our sleep and sex drive as well. In some individuals, thirst can sometimes masquerade as hunger. The next time you get the urge to grab that bag of potato chips, you may actually need a glass of water. If you want to figure out if your thirst and hunger sensations match up, do the following:

- When you feel hungry or have the need to snack, drink a large glass of water.
- If the hunger sensation does not go away or stops initially, but then returns within ten to twenty minutes, then it is most likely hunger and not thirst.
- If the hunger sensation stops after drinking water and does not return, then it was thirst, and you had your thirst sensation confused for hunger.

4: The Type of Water You Drink Also Makes a Difference

The best type of water is mineral enriched, such as purified spring or well water. The next best is filtered tap water. Water filtration systems employing activated carbon filters or reverse osmosis are good choices. I would avoid drinking distilled water. Since it is devoid of minerals, it is alleged to leech minerals from our bodies to balance itself out. If you are generally healthy and have a good diet with plenty of fruits and veggies, then it might not be a problem to drink distilled water, but I would still err on the side of caution.

Drinking tap water is also acceptable if the water is treated properly by the municipality you live in and is biologically safe to consume. If you are drinking tap water, run the cold water for a minute first thing in the morning to reduce lead contamination from solder joints in the pipes. Always drink cold water from the tap and never hot water. The hot-water system in your home may contaminate the water with unsafe impurities. If your tap water is chlorinated and you are not using any kind of chlorine filter, such as an activated carbon filter, then simply fill cool water in glass jugs and let it sit overnight to let the chlorine evaporate as much as possible. However, this is not a guaranteed method, and I would suggest investing in an inexpensive over-the-counter water filter for peace of mind.

5: What about Other Beverages?

Caffeinated beverages do not count completely toward your water requirements. They act as diuretics, making us urinate more and leading to a negative water balance (although your body does adapt to the caffeine and with time learns to preserve water). If you are a coffee or tea drinker, keep in mind that you may need to drink additional water to help preserve the water balance in your body. This is also true for caffeinated soft drinks, some of which have added salt. But don't feel bad every time you have that soft drink. My philosophy is everything in moderation. If you cannot enjoy the drink with your entire being, you might as well not drink it. The smarter way is to do it when it matters most, like in social gatherings and when you are more relaxed. Try green tea instead. Green tea is lower in caffeine and has more health benefits. Furthermore, if you are a juice drinker, limit your juice consumption to two cups a day, since juice is high in fructose, an excess of which is known to accumulate in the liver as fat. Most store brands for juice also have added artificial colors and flavors, which have their own adverse health effects. Go for fresh juice instead from a juice bar, or make the juice yourself at home.

6: How You Store Drinking Water Is Also Important

It's best to store water in glass containers. Another good choice is stainless steel. Avoid storing any liquids you consume in plastic bottles. If drinking from plastic bottles, make sure they are not left out in a hot car. Extreme temperatures will leach hormone-disrupting chemicals such as bisphenol A (BPA) from these plastic bottles, and these chemicals are not friendly to our bodies.[4] A better option for plastic bottles and containers may be the BPA-free versions. These containers use the bisphenol S (BPS) version of the chemical, which is thought to be less dangerous; however, a new study suggests that, at least in zebra fish, which share 80 percent of our DNA, low exposure to the BPS version of the chemical resulted in similar neural development issues as when exposed to BPA.[5] The long-term health effects of BPA-free plastic is unknown, so use it with caution. Having said all that, if you use plastic water bottles regularly, don't worry. Gradually try to use them less, while switching to glass or stainless steel bottles. Eventually, keep plastic bottled water for emergency use only.

7: Shower Rules

Hot, chlorinated water can harm the skin and lungs through long-term exposure. The hotter the water, the greater the damage. Unless you invest in a shower filter that removes chlorine, keep hot-water showers short, under ten minutes. You are not trying to poach yourself. Furthermore, during long, hot showers, you can sweat a lot unknowingly, which can dehydrate you. This may become an issue if you already have unregulated low blood pressure, as you could get dizzy or faint and hurt yourself. Also, by using less hot water, you are saving yourself money from reduced energy bills.

Keep the bathroom exhaust fan on while you take a shower to minimize breathing in the chlorine and other volatile organic compounds released from the steam. A better option would be to shower with warm or lukewarm water, just hot enough for you to feel the heat.

8: How Much Water to Consume

How much water you need to keep well hydrated and to keep your metabolism strong is not fixed, and the general rule of drinking eight glasses of water does not apply to everyone. Requirements will change with the level of physical activity, age, gender, sweating, breathing, urination, stool hardness, metabolism, and many other biological factors. Although drinking water is an important aspect of good health, other sources of water are just as important. During digestion, the body absorbs water in fruits and vegetables, and many other foods will hydrate us to some level. We may not always have access to clean drinking water, such as when we travel. In such situations, hydrating through water-rich foods like melons, grapefruits, oranges, cucumbers, celery, and tomatoes may be a good option.[6]

In general, men need more fluids (water plus beverages) than women. Men need on average three liters per day, whereas women need to consume 2.2 liters per day. Pregnant women need slightly more, and lactating women need to consume as much water as men.[7] These are just guidelines and should be taken as such. As we learned earlier, let your thirst and the color of your urine be a guide to how much water you need, and you should be well hydrated.

9: When to Drink Water Also Makes a Difference

We get dehydrated when we sleep through respiration and other metabolic processes. Therefore, when you wake up in the morning, before brushing your teeth, drink two to three (250 ml) cups of room-temperature to lukewarm water. Have your breakfast after half an hour. This should give you enough time to get ready for your day and for your stomach to absorb the water. Also, half an hour before lunch and dinner, drink one to two cups of water. This will improve your digestion and help you feel fuller faster.

If you are constipated or have weak digestion, squeeze half a lemon or lime into a cup of lukewarm water and drink that a couple of times in the day, preferably fifteen to twenty minutes before your main meals of the day. It will help stimulate production of gastric juices in the stomach and bile from the liver, which acts as a laxative. If you notice teeth sensitivity when drinking lemon/lime water, then drink through a straw to protect your teeth.

Try not to drink any water with food and for one hour after eating. That includes other drinks as well. Drinking large amounts of fluids with food will dilute your digestive enzymes and possibly impair your digestion. You may sip small amounts of water with your meals, especially if consuming dry foods. This suggestion may go against what you are used to, and there may be resistance to changing this behavior. If you are generally well hydrated and have good digestion, then I would not worry as much about the timing of water consumption.

If you follow the suggestions here, then you will be adequately hydrated throughout the day and experience some or all of the following health benefits:

- Your digestion will improve.
- You will manage your weight more effectively.
- Your skin will feel more supple and resilient.
- Your mind will be sharp and focused, with fewer headaches.
- Your kidneys will function optimally.
- You will feel energized throughout your day.[8]

10: The Wonderful World of Hydrotherapy

Hydrotherapy is the application of water at different temperatures to the body to elicit a healing response. One of the main modalities of naturopathic medicine when it first originated in North America was hydrotherapy. Hydrotherapy works by improving or normalizing blood flow, since it was believed that poor circulation leads to poor health. Currently, one of the leading uses of hydrotherapy is in recovering from injury and pain conditions, such as arthritis and low back pain.[9]

Although hydrotherapy can be used to treat several health conditions, I will introduce you to it through a powerful and simple technique that you can do by yourself. It is called a contrast shower (or alternating hot and cold showers). This is a whole-body treatment that will boost your metabolism, supercharge your immune system, reduce inflammation, and make you feel great overall.[10] The best way to do this therapy is at the end of your normal shower routine, after you have cleansed your body. Start with three minutes of warm water or as hot as you can handle, followed by one minute of cool water or as cold as you can handle. Repeat the hot and cold process at least two more times. Make sure to hit large body areas such as the upper and middle back, chest, stomach, and thighs, and ensure that the ambient room temperature during and after the shower is warm and not cold. If you are in a rush, one sixty-second cold blast at the end of your shower is a quick version of this method. The trick is to always end on "cold" so that the increased circulation removes toxins that have been mobilized by the heat.

It is believed that the heat from the shower dilates the capillaries under our skin. This will increase blood flow, and the sudden cooling that follows contracts the capillaries, sending a rush of blood inward toward large detoxifying organs such as the liver and kidneys. It may be hard initially to do the whole minute of cold shower. If that is the case, you can start with sixty seconds of warm and twenty seconds of cool and build up from there as your tolerance improves, always keeping the 3:1 ratio between hot and cold. New research shows that exposure to a cold environment over time can activate and increase brown fat activity (brown fat is a more metabolically active fat), allowing us to burn off more calories.[11]

A note of caution: individuals with acute skin infections, peripheral neuropathy, seizures, hypotension, Raynaud's disease, and severe cardiac complications should avoid doing this therapy or do it under a doctor's supervision.[12]

11: Simple Ways to Save Water

Water preservation is something we humans should all be concerned about. The world has a limited supply of drinkable water, and this limited resource is diminishing every day. If you live somewhere with unrestricted access to clean water, then consider yourself fortunate. Many people in the developing world still have trouble accessing clean drinking water. So what can you do that is not as extreme as going on a water-conservation crusade? Below are simple suggestions anyone can do to help preserve one of our most precious resources.

- Simply being aware of the need to preserve water is the first step. From the time you wake up to the time you sleep, think of the ways you use water and how you could waste less.
- When you brush your teeth, if you have the habit of leaving the tap open, make a conscious effort to close the tap for the two minutes you are brushing your teeth. For individuals who shave, the same rule applies. Instead of running the tap, fill a small bowl with water to clean the razor.
- If you use a dishwasher, then try to use it when it's full of dirty dishes and not when it's less than half full. My preference is to wash the dishes by hand and air-dry them. I give a quick sprinkle of water

and then apply the soap with the tap closed. Then I quickly wash the dishes using the rubbing force of my hands.

- While bathing, if you can turn the shower off while you use soap or shampoo, then make it a habit to do that. All those short intervals will add up to significant savings. My personal strategy is to use one of those kitchen egg timers and set it for seven minutes to limit my shower time. When I know I have a fixed amount of time to clean myself, I become more efficient and daydream less during showers. Maybe this is a strategy you can use during the weekdays. Then on weekends you can have longer, warmer showers or baths to relax.

- Doing laundry is a necessity, but that doesn't mean we do it every day or every other day. Most modern washing machines are high efficiency and use less water, which is good. If you don't already have one, consider upgrading. Also, if you are not already doing so, try to do laundry just once a week and fill the machine to full capacity. Reconsider what dirty clothes mean to you. If you are indoors most of the time, how dirty do your clothes actually get? The clothing items touching genitals and armpits tend to smell more because of the oils released by the sebaceous glands there. I would wash those items regularly; however, other clothing items are a judgment call. Use your sense of smell and sight and not mere habit to decide what needs to be washed.

- Outside the house, there are areas where we can save water as well. Water depletion can happen from watering plants. To reduce the need to water the plants often, consider planting floras native to your area. Such indigenous plants are generally more drought resistant and require less upkeep.

- Consider using barrels to collect rainwater coming down the roof of your home. This water can be used later for watering your plants during times of drought. It's an easy DIY project and there are tons of videos on YouTube that show you how to do it. Just a note of caution: there may be restrictions with your municipality, so check for any such restrictions before embarking on this project.

- Washing cars is something some of us do often, while others do it only when necessary. Realize your car-washing habits, and try to wash your car only when needed.

- One last area where we can save water as consumers is in a hidden source of water use. Any guesses? It's actually eating meat. Raising animals for their meat uses a lot of water, much more than growing plants for food. One source puts the average amount of water used to raise one pound of beef at eighteen hundred gallons, which is equivalent to 90 eight-minute-long showers.[13,14] That is approximately three months' worth of showers if you shower daily. Comparatively, it takes about 108 gallons of water to produce a pound of a vegetable like corn.[15] It's mind-boggling and humbling to know how much water we use and where our water resources go. Having learned this, if you eat meat on a regular basis, I don't expect you to give it up. But you might consider eating it less often, knowing that you will be saving a precious resource. This may take some time, but fewer people eating meat will eventually translate to fewer animals raised and more water saved.

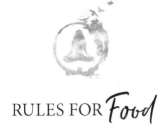

RULES FOR *Food*

Healthy eating is not about dieting or restricting major food groups; it's about lifestyle choices, reengineering our eating habits, and self-discovery. If you consider your digestive system as a furnace, then the fire in it is what burns your food to create the energy you need. Some people have this furnace set on high and burn through food quickly, and some are set on low and it takes them longer. People burn calories at different rates. It may seem unfair that some people can eat whatever they want and not gain a single ounce, while someone else will smell a doughnut and gain five pounds. A calorie is not a calorie to everyone. Therefore, just restricting calories is not a smart way to lose or maintain a healthy weight. Giving our bodies the nutrients they need is more important than counting calories. We have to understand our body's needs and incorporate a holistic approach of healthier food choices.

Food fuels our bodies and provides it with nutrients to repair itself, grow, and fight diseases. There are macronutrients like carbohydrates, proteins, and fats, and then there are micronutrients like vitamins and minerals. All your nutritional needs can be attained from foods alone, provided you eat a wide variety of whole, unprocessed foods. Many diets promise to give you the body you want, but research has not conclusively proven that one is better than the other. One of the most profound influences you can have on your health is to pay attention to the food you are eating and choose it wisely. I will try my best to help you in this endeavor with my recommendations below. Use the tools presented in this chapter to create your own perfectly balanced diet.

1: Meat, Poultry, and Fish in Moderation

Meat is not bad if it is unprocessed and consumed in moderation. Red meat from commercial factory farms is considered unhealthy, especially if it's cured and processed into deli meats and sausages. Because of their high cholesterol, salt, and nitrite contents, their consumption over time has been linked to heart disease, diabetes,[1] and stomach cancer.[2] Healthier choices of meat would be meat from poultry and fish. Toxins tend to accumulate in the meat of these animals, mainly depending on the quality of food they eat throughout their life cycle—and since a larger animal will eat more, it accumulates a larger toxic load. In general, when consuming meat, go for meats from smaller animals to minimize the toxic load entering your body.

If red meat forms most of your diet, then try to get it from cows that are exclusively pasture raised and grass fed throughout their life, as they are more nutritious and have a lower toxic load. For poultry meat and eggs, go for free range or organic.

When choosing fish, go for the acronym SMASH (salmon, mackerel, anchovies, sardines, and herring). These fish have lower mercury content and should be safe to consume in moderate quantities. Eat two to three servings of fish a week to get beneficial fish oils rich in omega-3s (eicosapentaenoic acid [EPA] and docosahexaenoic acid [DHA]), which are known to help with heart and brain health. A serving of meat is typically the size of a deck of cards. Larger fishes like shark, tuna, and swordfish tend to be higher in mercury, so try to avoid them, or at least minimize their consumption. Some commercial fishes are grown in fish farms under deplorable conditions and are fed high-fat processed feeds to make them fat fast. Because of the high-density populations in these fish farms, disease can be common, requiring antibiotics. Although farmed salmon are a good source of healthy omega-3 fatty acids, they can contain high concentrations of polychlorinated biphenyls (PCBs), dioxins, and chlorinated pesticides.[3] If possible, choose wild-caught fish instead. Depending on where you live, eating wild-caught fish can get expensive. If all you can afford is farm-raised fish, then try to find out the pollution level of the waters the fish were bred in to minimize ingesting the organochlorine compounds found in these fish. However, the benefit of eating farmed fatty fish like salmon will still outweigh the risk associated with eating it. Some folks cannot tolerate the smell or taste of fish. In such cases, getting your fish oil from supplements in the form of a capsule may be ideal. I would recommend getting between 500 and 1,000 mg of combined EPA and DHA daily to maintain good health. Look for ones derived from molecularly distilled fish oils and independently tested to be free of heavy metals such as mercury and lead. Take your fish oil capsules while eating food, in the beginning or middle of your meal, to minimize any fishy burp or aftertaste that can happen. Alternatively, you can look for odorless fish oil products and try different brands until you find one that you are happy with. If you are on anticoagulant drugs such as Coumadin (warfarin), use extra caution taking fish oil, as it can affect blood clotting. Let your doctor know, as dosages may need to be adjusted to reach your international normalized ratio (INR) target.

2: Choose More Vegetables

On the whole, a vegetarian diet is a healthier option for you and the planet. Vegetarians tend to live longer, have fewer cardiovascular events, and maintain healthier weights than people who consume a meat-based diet.[4] Considering the importance of vegetables, they should take up half your plate during any meal. Green leafy vegetables, especially the darker variety, are high in calcium, vitamin K, and other nutrients, and they should be indulged in often, as they help your body detox efficiently. Frozen or canned vegetables are also a good option for people who don't always have access to fresh vegetables. They tend to have high nutritional content, as they are canned or frozen within hours after harvest. Discussing which vegetables are the best to eat for specific health benefits would fill another book. I suggest that you find yourself at least a dozen or so vegetables that you enjoy eating. Eat a rainbow of colors to ensure you are consuming a varied amount of nutrients, and you will have most of your bases covered. As long as you eat healthy 80 percent of the time, consider yourself on the right track, and don't get upset with yourself if you indulge once in a while.

3: Where to Buy Your Groceries

When it comes to fruits and vegetables, it's best to get them from local farms or go organic. Check out ewg.org for the Dirty Dozen, which are the top twelve most highly polluted fruits and vegetables. At the time of this writing, they are strawberries, spinach, nectarines, apples, grapes, peaches, cherries, pears, tomatoes, celery, potatoes, and sweet bell peppers.[5] Get these organic if you can. The Environmental Working Group (EWG) also has a Clean Fifteen list of the least polluted fruits and vegetables. These are avocados, sweet corn, pineapples, cabbages, onions, frozen sweet peas, papayas, asparagus, mangoes, eggplants, honeydew melon, kiwis, cantaloupes, cauliflower, and broccoli. The EWG has highlighted that a small amount of sweet corn, papaya, and summer squash sold in the United States is produced from genetically modified seeds. They recommend getting organic varieties of these crops if you want to avoid genetically modified produce.[6]

Producing high-yield crops has been made possible by using synthetic pesticides, herbicides, and fertilizers. Due to the farming practices in the last few decades, the same crop is grown year after year on the same soil. Because of this practice, certain nutrients have been depleted from the soil and hence from the food you are eating. But I am happy to see that more and more farms are adopting the traditional practice of rotating crops and using integrated pest management to keep pest population under control while minimizing use of chemical pesticides.[7]

Have you ever noticed that when you bring certain fruits home from the supermarket, they can sit on your shelf, sometimes for weeks, without rotting? As you may have realized, depending on where you live, most produce travels a long distance, especially in winter, before getting to its final destination. That means most of these fruits are picked raw and still don't have their enzymes activated, something that would happen if they matured naturally. These enzymes are what ripen the fruits, releasing the full taste as well as making the nutrients more bioavailable. Buy local farm fruits and vegetables in season and see how fast they will ripen. Not only that, they taste much better and are more nutritious.[8]

Try to get to know your local farmers and their farming practices and support them by joining their food-distribution programs. Those of us who live in big cities can make use of farmers' markets, where local farmers sell their produce. Be aware that some vendors pretend to be farmers but are resellers who buy their produce from wholesalers. Some easy ways to figure out the good guys from the fraudsters is looking at what they sell. If a vegetable or fruit is of uniform size and shape, like you would find in a supermarket, then they are most likely resellers. Also, if you find produce sold out of season, like zucchini in April, then you know they are not local crops.

Buying local can get expensive. So if you are on a tight budget, it is okay to buy your groceries from the supermarket as long as you are aware that you may not be getting enough nutrition out of them. To offset this, buy produce in season from the supermarket that is sourced from a closer vicinity. Most supermarkets label their produce, declaring where it was grown. A great resource for finding out what's in season is seasonalfoodguide.org. Select the state you live in, and it will show you which fruits and veggies are in season for each month of the year.

If you have a small plot of land or access to a community garden and are so inclined, grow some of your own food. You will be amazed at how little space it takes to grow enough nutritious food for your family. You may look for community gardens in your neighborhood through communitygarden.org. This practice may help offset the high cost of buying organic produce and save money from not needing to buy supplements for you and your family. You can invest in a nice composter and use your family's food scraps to make high-quality fertilizer for your crops. For city dwellers who live in apartments, you can section off a sunny part of your balcony and grow veggies such as tomatoes, peppers, radishes, and lettuce. If you don't have a balcony, you could invest in a large window box or even grow herbs such as mint, parsley, and chives indoors in pots or mason jars or in dirt-free contraptions like the AeroGarden.

4: Nutritional Supplements Dos and Don'ts

I generally don't recommend supplements to my patients unless they are severely depleted or trying to treat a health concern. It's important to understand that taking a high enough dose of anything, even if it's nature derived, can be harmful if not done properly. Dosing on supplements is intricate and requires professional training. Dosing guidelines on the bottle are generally considered safe, but to get therapeutic dosing individualized to your physiology requires you to see a professional, such as a naturopath. If you suffer from any ailments or are taking medications, then consult a professional before taking any supplements to make sure there will be no adverse reactions.

Food-derived supplements are generally more bioavailable than synthetics, but they are pricier. If you can afford them, go for it. When choosing supplements, I would not go for the cheapest or the most expensive. You do pay a price for quality ingredients, up to a point. Read labels carefully. Most supplements will have fillers, binders, flow agents, and other excipients. They will be listed under the "other ingredient" section. These are things used to keep the tablet's shape and fill up space and perform other processes. In general, they are considered safe, but recently some of these excipients (titanium dioxide,[9] carrageenan,[10,11] and paraben[12]) have come under scrutiny, and there are questions as to their safety. Until the powers that be sort this out, choose products with as little fillers, binders, and other excipients as you can and you are golden. The cheaper products generally have more of these. Another way to minimize getting these in your supplements is to go for a liquid- or powder-based form instead of a tablet form. There are companies dedicated to having little to no fillers or binders in their products, so just search Google for excipient-free supplements and look for supplements you have access to.

If your family eats a typical American diet with a higher meat and junk-food consumption, coupled with fewer vegetables and fruits, then as a backup to your diet it might be beneficial to have a multivitamin/mineral supplement. Most multis are well formulated and have all the vitamins, including A, the Bs, C, D, E, and K, plus a range of minerals, including calcium, magnesium, zinc, copper, chromium, manganese, selenium, and molybdenum. Choose the top three multivitamins based on user reviews and take them on a rotating basis to ensure you get all the micronutrients your body may be missing. Some manufacturers consider your age and gender and have slightly different formulations based on those parameters. However, the main difference is usually the inclusion of iron. If you are a menstruating female or normally have low iron (ferritin) levels, then consider the multi with iron and check your blood iron levels regularly, every three months or so, to make sure your levels are going up. If not, you may need to try a different formulation. If you are on multiple medications, then take your multi a few hours away from your meds to prevent possible interactions. Taking a supplement is not an excuse to continue eating junk food. Try to eat a balanced diet as best you can.

At the end of the day, we have to weigh the pros and cons. Does the benefit of taking the supplement outweigh the possible risk associated with the excipients used in it? How much active ingredient is there in the product, and how bioavailable is it? These questions are why I advocate getting your nutrition from quality food made by Mother Nature. Over thousands of years, our bodies have developed an inherent intelligence to digest and extract exactly what is needed from the fruits and vegetables grown naturally. Embrace this intelligence and trust in it. Listen to your body, and it won't let you down.

5: Pick Protein Wisely

Protein is your friend. It boosts your metabolism, helps to build and repair tissue and make hormones and assist in a multitude of processes within the body. However, more is not always better, and the type of protein makes a difference. Animal protein is harder on your system. It takes a considerable amount of digestive enzymes and energy to digest it. As a solution, consume animal protein with some lime/lemon or apple cider vinegar in a little water to help your body digest the meat better. Milk-based protein such as whey may be a better option, especially for those who want to put on muscle mass, as it stimulates protein synthesis.[13] Some people are sensitive to casein, the other major protein found in milk, or are lactose intolerant. For such individuals, plant-based protein may be a better option. If going for powder-based plant protein, a combination product that uses two or more types of protein is always better than a single protein source. Some common vegetarian protein sources are beans, tofu, nut butters, tempeh, quinoa, hemp, peas, lentils, chickpeas, nuts, and seeds.

6: Eat a Handful of Nuts and Seeds as a Snack

Nuts and seeds are high in good-quality fats and proteins, which will keep you satiated and help control your cravings. They are also a good source of omega-3 oils, which are good for heart and brain health.[14,15] Make nuts like walnuts, almonds, and pistachios part of your daily diet, in moderation. I consider these to be guilt-free snacks. I don't snack often, but when I do, I grab a handful of nuts and munch slowly; it keeps me full for quite some time. Seeds like flax and chia[16] are also high in omega-3s and are good to make a part of your diet, as they can keep your cholesterol in check.[17] You can add a couple tablespoons of flax to your morning porridge or yogurt or any other dish you like. Chia seeds can expand considerably, so make sure that happens outside your body. The seeds should dissolve in your food, not in your throat. Letting them sit for fifteen to twenty minutes in a liquid medium should do the trick. You may also choose to soak a couple tablespoons of chia seeds overnight in a glass of water and drink or eat them in the morning as a breakfast substitute. This can be quite satiating and will produce amazing bowel movements. As with implementing any dietary changes, start with a small amount and build from there. For example, with chia seeds, start with one teaspoon for the first three days, increasing by a teaspoon each time until you reach two tablespoons, which is equivalent to six teaspoons. Observe how your body reacts to any dietary changes. Initially there may be digestive disturbances or energy fluctuations, but that should settle down. If it doesn't, then stop eating that food. If the food you are eating is compatible with your physiology, you will feel no difference or better than before. All foods may not suit you; don't force yourself to eat something just because it's considered healthy. It needs to be right for you.

7: Plant Fat v. Animal Fat

Animal fats have a bad reputation, especially when cooked for a long time over high heat, as with a grill. This leads to the creation of carcinogenic compounds, which have the potential to cause cancer.[18,19] If you love to barbecue, marinate the meat longer using a vinegar base with turmeric and garlic, and use herbs like mint, rosemary, and thyme. Cook over a low to medium flame, making sure the meat doesn't burn. If you can, prevent the fat drippings from incomplete combustion. This seems to reduce the release of smoke containing the toxic polycyclic aromatic hydrocarbons (PAHs) that can seep into the meat.[20]

If the animal fat you consume comes from grass-fed or organically grown animals, then eating this fat in moderation is ideal. Plant-based fats are a healthier option. Some of the good plant fats come from coconuts, avocados, olives, nuts, and seeds. Olive oil, which forms the foundation of the Mediterranean diet, is considered a healthy option and should form part of your diet, in moderation. The more virgin the oil, the more delicate it is. To preserve its health benefits, olive and other virgin oils should not be exposed to heat. Heating oil for a long time will oxidize it and make it unhealthy. If frying, pick healthy oils that have a higher smoking point, such as grapeseed, avocado, or coconut oil. It's best to consume a diverse range of healthy oils to get all the different lengths and permutations of fatty acids. However, I would avoid corn, soy, and canola oil, since most of them are made from genetically modified organisms (GMOs) using toxic processes.[21]Although omega-3 oils have received a lot of attention in recent years for their health benefits (and rightly so), there needs to be a balance between the different omega oils we consume, and more omega-3 is not necessarily better.

8: Probiotics 101

Probiotics are the beneficial bacteria that live in your gut. These outnumber the cells in your body by a ratio of ten to one, and they perform vital roles. They mainly reside in the large intestine and toward the end of the small intestine. Their job is to digest any remaining undigested food and release nutrients like vitamin B_{12}, vitamin K_2, and other amino acids for you to absorb.[22,23] They also release neurotransmitter molecules that will keep you in a good mood and cytokines that strengthen the immune system. Probiotics have also been shown to reduce incidents of inflammation and arthritis and modulate the effects of food allergies and eczema in children.[24,25] When you feed on junk food and lots of sugar, your gut flora get starved of the food they thrive on, preventing them from doing their job properly, and then they die off. This leaves room for bad bacteria, yeast, and fungi to flourish, and these wreak havoc on your system.

How do you make sure the good bacteria survive and flourish? Give them prebiotics (the food they like) and probiotics (a fresh supply of good bacteria). Prebiotics are mainly found in fiber-rich foods, like oats, beans, berries, nuts, seeds, and vegetables. Probiotics are naturally found in fermented foods, such as yogurt, kefir, miso, natto, tempeh, sauerkraut, kimchi, pickles, and kombucha. If you are sensitive to dairy, nondairy options of yogurt and kefir are available. Incorporate more fiber-rich food into your diet, and slowly increase your probiotic food intake to prevent the production of excess gas, which can happen if you suddenly increase your intake. Some fermented foods may not agree with you and give you digestive difficulties such as stomach ache or diarrhea. If these symptoms don't subside within a few days, then stop eating that food. Try different varieties to figure out which fermented foods are compatible with your gut.

Preferably, you should eat probiotic-rich foods like the fermented foods mentioned above, but if you can't, then taking a multistrain probiotic supplement with a minimum of 5 to 10 billion cfu on a regular basis is a good measure for keeping a healthy gut. Just be careful. As with fermented foods, some probiotics may not suit you and can create digestive issues. You may have to try a few before settling on one that you like. If you are immune compromised, then don't take a probiotic unless under the supervision of a doctor. Moreover, don't take probiotics when you are constipated. Make sure you are having regular bowel movements while taking probiotics.

9: Sugar Is Your Nemesis

Sugar is sneaky, and it hides everywhere. Most processed, prepackaged, ready-made foods, pastries, and drinks are loaded with high-fructose corn syrup, an excess of which our bodies will immediately store as fat. Plus, this sweetener has mercury contamination, which is currently unregulated.[26]

Consuming grain products like bread, rice, pasta, and cereals on a regular basis may lead to weight gain. Most of these products are highly refined and made of simple carbs, which will raise your blood sugar levels, leading to a rise in insulin and storage of these molecules as triglycerides (fat). Complex carbs found in vegetables will digest steadily, giving a slower release of glucose, making them a better source of carbs.

Always watch out for the sugar content of any product you purchase, and choose products with the lowest sugar content. If one of the first three ingredients listed is sugar or any of its alternatives, such as sucrose or fructose, then I would suggest putting that product back on the shelf and choosing a healthier option. If you must use a sweetener, then avoid artificial sweeteners like aspartame and saccharin and go for the real deal. Use stevia, raw honey, coconut sugar, or maple syrup.

10: How You Eat Your Food Makes a Difference

The stomach releases hydrochloric acid and other gastric juices to kill pathogens (disease-causing organisms) commonly found on food and to digest your food. The better the food gets digested, the smaller the molecules become and the easier it is for your gut to absorb them.

- The stomach's main job is to digest proteins. Proteins take time to digest; therefore, they provide the most satiety, so include some form of protein with every meal.
- Starches and fats get digested mainly in the small intestine. Try not to combine proteins with simple starches like rice, bread, or pasta, because they will sit in the stomach and ferment, releasing gasses until they reach the small intestine. However, it's okay to eat vegetables with meats.
- Always eat fruits alone, away from other foods, because they digest fast. To minimize indigestion, eat sour fruits such as oranges and grapefruit separately from sweet fruits such as bananas and apples.
- The more fiber a food has, the better your digestion. Eat plenty of vegetables, which also come with their own digestive enzymes—an added bonus. If you want to implement more fiber-rich foods into your diet, do it gradually to allow your digestive system time to acclimatize, as you may produce more gas initially.

The act of eating also makes a big difference on how you digest your food.

Here are some important rules to follow:

- You have probably heard this many times, but it's important to chew your food thoroughly. By breaking down food in your mouth using the grinding action of your teeth, you are helping to expose a larger surface area of the food to the digestive enzymes in your gut, which will improve the digestion and absorption of nutrients. If you are eating an entire plate of food in less than ten minutes, slow it down to twenty minutes.
- It is important for you to be relaxed while eating your meals. When relaxed, your body goes into the parasympathetic mode (the rest and relaxation mode). Blood will be directed to the digestive system,

which will allow you to digest your meals more efficiently and maximize nutrient absorption. Therefore, when you are in a hurry or anxious, don't eat. Eating in such a state may give you indigestion. When you have time to eat, close your eyes and take a few slow, deep breaths. When you feel a sense of calm within, your body is ready to accept food.

- Try not to watch TV while eating. If you do watch, go for shows that will lift your mood and not ones that will depress you or make you anxious. As an alternative, listen to some light instrumental music or any music that relaxes you and puts you in the parasympathetic mode.

- Try to eat most of your meals while seated at a table, or at least do this for the biggest meal of the day. Sit at a table and look at your food and enjoy the smell and taste. Your focus should be on your meal and nothing else. You may have light, pleasant conversations when eating with others, but nothing too distracting or emotional. Try not to think of eating as a chore that needs to get done. It should be a pleasurable activity, a time to unwind, relax, and take in sustenance.

- The aim of all these suggestions is to help you be in a relaxed state while eating, which will minimize indigestion and maximize nutrient absorption. You don't have to do everything mentioned, but adapt what you can to suit your lifestyle.

11: You Are What You Absorb

For a long time, the popular notion was, "You are what you eat." Now we have come to realize that absorption is just as important. Depending on how efficient one's digestive system is, a nutritious meal for one person may not provide the nutrient requirements for someone else because of poor absorption.

You can think of your digestive system as a tube that starts from the mouth and ends at the anus. The inside of this tube is technically considered an external environment, even though it resides inside your body. Your immune system needs to protect you from invaders from the external environment; hence, a large part of your immunity resides close to your digestive system. It monitors everything being absorbed by the gut lining, and if something doesn't look right, it will try to sequester and destroy it.

A lifetime of food sensitivities and intolerances can damage the gut lining and prevent uptake of essential nutrients, leading to a cascade of health failures. Consuming the same food over and over again and eating highly processed foods with artificial ingredients may be the culprits. For individuals who have difficulty absorbing certain nutrients, supplementation may be necessary until your gut heals. If you have multiple sensitivities to many different foods and you experience joint stiffness and pain, headaches, fatigue, rashes, chronic diarrhea, or constipation, then you may have advanced to leaky gut syndrome or intestinal hyperpermeability, where the tight junctions within your intestinal lining malfunction. This allows undigested food particles and bacteria to leak into the bloodstream and create systemic immune reactions, which can create widespread inflammation and pain within the body.[27] If you suspect you have this, you may benefit from working with a professional, such as a naturopath, to figure out how to resolve this condition.

12: Keep a Food Journal

If you notice lots of gas or heartburn after a meal, most likely you are not digesting it well. Either you are not producing enough digestive enzymes or are sensitive to certain foods. Keep a food journal to help you identify which foods or additives are the culprit. Note what you eat at a particular time and observe how you feel for the next few hours. When you feel any symptoms, note them. If you do get symptoms, take a break from eating that food group for a couple of days, and then eat it again and see what happens. This is a simple way of figuring out which foods you are intolerant to. It can be a challenge, but once you know and eliminate the offending foods from your diet, you will feel much better. Alcohol, chocolates, deep-fried foods, and spicy foods are the common culprits for heartburn. Also, starving yourself and then consuming a large amount of food can give you heartburn. Bowel movements are a good indicator of how good your digestion is. A well-formed soft stool that holds its shape is good. Stools that are loose with froth most likely indicate food sensitivities and inflammation in the gut. A hard stool that is difficult to pass may indicate a lack of fluids or fiber in the diet. As for color, different shades of brown are normal. If you are consistently seeing any other color, such as black, yellow, green, or brownish red, get medical attention. Ideally, you would pass a stool for every major meal, but even once a day is good.

13: Going Vegan

I would recommend not going completely off animal protein unless you educate yourself on vegetarian sources of protein and a vegan lifestyle. If you have been eating meat your whole life, going full vegan (no meat, eggs, or dairy products) will be a shock to your system. Your gut enzymes and bacteria have adjusted themselves to accepting meat. It will take time for your gut to reeducate itself on the change in your food choices. You may have to supplement nutrients like vitamin B_{12} and iron until your diet is sorted out. Join a vegan support group or get the support of like-minded individuals who have had success in the transition. Growing children have higher nutritional requirements; therefore, I would advise against them going vegan. In my practice, I have seen patients going vegan after seeing a documentary, only to end up in my office with nutritional deficiencies and health issues.

I am not trying to discourage you from adopting a vegan lifestyle. It is totally doable and a very healthy lifestyle, but it can be a challenge to maintain long term, especially if you don't have a good support system and are not well educated on it. My goal here is to help you make lifestyle choices that are healthy and sustainable. If you eat meat, then my recommendation is to be vegetarian about 70 percent of the time and eat animal products 30 percent of the time, which will translate to eating good-quality meat two days a week and a vegetarian diet the remaining five days. If you are a vegetarian and it's working for you, then keep doing what you are doing. If it's not working for you, look at your protein sources and expand on those, as that is usually the weak link in the diet.

14: More Helpful Tips

- Make a healthy diet part of your lifestyle, and introduce small habits that are sustainable. Slow and steady always wins the race.
- When shopping for groceries, don't go when you're hungry. You will most likely buy more junk food. Before shopping, if you are hungry and cannot eat a meal, eat a small, protein-rich snack, such as a handful of almonds.
- Shop on the store's perimeter, where healthier options such as fruits and vegetables are located.
- When buying prepackaged foods, always read the labels. If there are a lot of big, scientific-sounding words on the ingredients list, it may not be something you want to eat. These types of highly processed foods with artificial flavors, colors, and preservatives are not inherently bad, but our bodies are not designed to work with them. Our digestive system has evolved to process fruits, vegetables, and animal meat. The sudden introduction of these novel food items is sometimes more than your system can handle.
- At home, put fruit out in a bowl in high-traffic areas. If it's seen and looks appetizing, it's more likely to be eaten.
- Eat two to three main meals and use smaller plates if you are trying to lose weight. You don't have to eat snacks. Give your digestive system a break, and it will thank you. Eating small meals throughout the day can exhaust your pancreas, which has to constantly pump out insulin to manage the blood sugar within an acceptable range and store the excess as fat. Furthermore, since the body is used to acquiring energy from an external source every two to three hours, it doesn't rely on

internal fat reserves for energy, which can make it difficult to lose weight.

- Use different herbs and spices when cooking; they will make the food tastier and easier to digest. You also won't need as much salt.
- Try to cook food at home as much as possible instead of eating out. Restaurants tend to use more oil, salt, and sugar in their dishes. However, there is a growing trend of health-conscious eateries offering wholesome and tasty food choices.
- When cooking food at home, use single-ingredient products as much as possible and cook foods from scratch instead of relying on ready-made foods that you just heat and serve.
- Be more aware of where your food comes from, and choose more locally grown foods. Buy foods in season and select quality over quantity.

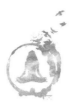

RULES FOR *Sleep*

Lack of sleep has become an epidemic in our time. As a society, we have gone from valuing a good night's rest to valuing how much we can get done while awake. The advances in electronic devices have not made getting a good night's rest any easier. People are glued to their screens everywhere you look, and all that mental stimulation is keeping us more awake than ever. With the stresses of modern life and everyone's hectic schedules, one can argue that the older times were simpler times and that there wasn't much stress, so people could sleep peacefully. This may be partially true, but we must adapt to our time, and it all comes down to personal choices and prioritizing things that are important to you.

Although productivity is what makes us advance, cutting back on sleep is not the way to go. A good night's rest is just as important as good-quality food or clean air and water. Most people focus on how much you need to sleep, but how well you sleep is equally important. We need time to get into those deep stages of sleep, where most of the restorative and healing functions happen.

It may interest you to know that sleeping less has been independently associated with being overweight.[1,2] It reduces the satiety hormone leptin and increases our appetite stimulator hormone ghrelin, which increases our hunger, especially for carb-rich foods, and this can lead to weight gain.[3] Observe yourself the next time you don't get a good night's rest. Do you crave high-sugar or high-fat foods? Studies also show that sleeping less than seven to eight hours increases your risk of coronary heart disease and stroke.[4] That may explain why most heart attacks happen on Mondays. The added stress of going back to work, combined with sleeping less, may be the triggers.

Another important area where sleep plays a role is in immunity. Even a partial night of sleep deprivation reduces natural killer and cellular immune responses in humans.[5] Furthermore, higher rates of depression are reported by individuals with sleep disorders involving insomnia and obstructive sleep apnea.[6] We are just beginning to graze the surface of the importance of sleep, and there is much that we have yet to discover. We spend a third of our lives sleeping. If you could think of having good-quality sleep as keeping a high-interest, tax-free savings account, then you would make sure to keep that account topped up regularly, so the interest keeps adding up. Give your sleep the same importance you would give to your money, and watch the benefits add up.

1: Ideal Sleep Requirements

In general, adults require between seven and nine hours of sleep to stay healthy and function optimally.[7] How much sleep you need depends on your individual biochemical needs. The best way to figure this out is to do the following:

- Go to sleep nine hours before your intended wake time, and set your alarm for after nine hours. After a couple weeks of this routine, if you wake up before your alarm rings and feel rested, then that is how much sleep you require. If you wake up with the alarm and still feel unrested, then increase your sleep time to ten or eleven hours and see if that helps.
- If you are an adult who consistently needs more than ten hours of sleep to feel rested, then that is what you require; however, since this is out of the norm, there is most likely a medical issue, and you may need to bring this up with your doctor.

2: Melatonin's Effect on the Circadian Rhythm

Your sleep is regulated by your circadian rhythm, which is controlled by a tiny gland in your brain called the pineal gland. This gland relies on light and darkness as one of the main signals to release a sleep hormone, melatonin, that gives you the urge to sleep. Light inhibits the gland, and darkness activates it.[8] If your sleep patterns are all over the place, then do the following to restore them:

- When you first wake up, open the blinds and let in daylight to reset your pineal gland. This drops your melatonin to daytime levels.
- Try to get at least ten minutes of natural light daily to reset your clock. In the winter months, you can use full-spectrum lights to provide the same effect if it is cloudy.
- Don't take long naps in the daytime; if you must nap, make it no more than twenty minutes long.
- In the evening, as it gets closer to bedtime, lower the lights in the house to signal to your body that it's time to sleep. If possible, use light dimmers to keep the lights low.
- Make sure the room is cool and extremely dark when sleeping. Use blackout curtains, if needed, and cover all sources of light.
- If you wake up at night to urinate, use a nightlight instead of turning on the main lights. Use a red light for your nightlight, because it does not seem to interfere with sleep and may actually improve sleep quality, according to a study done with female atheletes.[9]

- Taking a shower or bath one to two hours before bed will heat up your core temperature. As your body cools, it will signal your pineal gland to release melatonin, which will help you to fall asleep quicker.[10]
- Trying to catch up on sleep on the weekends just dysregulates your circadian rhythm. Try to keep the same bedtime routine throughout the week. Go to bed by 11 p.m. at the latest to allow your stress glands (the adrenal glands) to recharge and rejuvenate.[11]
- Wear light, loose, and comfortable clothing to bed to allow the body to naturally cool at night, which allows the release of melatonin.

3: Ways to Minimize Sleep Disruption

People who experience sleep issues often overlook simple things that may cause them to miss out on the precious sleep they need.

- Just as light can inhibit sleep, noise can also interfere with sleep. Try to minimize sources of noise. Otherwise, use a white-noise machine to drown out the other noises. There are white-noise apps available as well.
- Avoid drinking fluids in the two to three hours before bed, especially if you tend to wake up at night to urinate. You may sip on a bit of water if you get thirsty. Be aware that alcohol in the evening may disrupt your sleep pattern and prevent you from reaching the deeper stages of sleep. How much alcohol it will take to interfere with your sleep depends on how well you metabolize it. Women generally get intoxicated faster than men because of how they metabolize and absorb alcohol.
- If you drink coffee, drink it in the morning or by noon at the latest. It takes hours for the caffeine to break down and clear away from your system, potentially interfering with your sleep if you are sensitive to caffeine.
- Pain is another reason people can't sleep well and get the deep, restful sleep they so desire. Usually it's the major joints that hurt because of the pressure of the body on them when we sleep. If you have a chronic pain condition, then learning to manage the pain properly is important. Relaxation techniques, such as deep breathing and progressive muscle relaxation, which I will talk about shortly, are helpful. Don't be reluctant to take pain medication to help you sleep, if that is your only choice. The benefit of restful sleep may outweigh the negative effects of the medication. Some people who have tried many things without relief have found acupuncture to be helpful. This traditional Chinese medicine is starting to show promise for many pain conditions.

- If you have shoulder pain, try to sleep on your back or on the side that doesn't hurt. If you are a side sleeper, you may benefit from a softer mattress and a thicker pillow. The goal is to keep the spine straight and aligned when sleeping to minimize pressure on it. Also, keep a pillow between your knees to ease the pressure on your hip joints.
- The worst position to sleep in is on your stomach. Sleeping on your belly puts pressure on your spine, flattening the curve and compressing your lower back the whole night, which will cause pain and stiffness. Furthermore, your neck will also suffer because of the twisted side placement, putting strain on the muscles and nerves in the area.

4: Low Blood Sugar Can Wake You Up

Generally, sleep between three and four hours after dinner. Going to bed on a full stomach can interfere with sleep and cause indigestion. On the flip side, going to bed hungry can also disrupt your sleep. If your last meal was more than five hours before bed, eat a light, protein-rich snack, such as a handful of nuts, an hour before bed. This will keep your blood sugar steady and prevent a middle-of-the-night cortisol spike, which can wake you up.

5: Minimize Screen Use before Bed

In today's fast-paced digital world of electronics and internet, our minds are overstimulated, and this stimulus sometimes prevents us from getting a good night's rest. Electronic devices like TVs, cell phones, tablets, and laptops will disrupt your pineal gland. The blue light from these screens, which is in the 460 nanometer range, interferes with melatonin release.[12] Avoid using them for the hour before bed. If you must use these devices before bed, make sure the screen brightness is set to the lowest level and minimize your exposure time. Blue-light screen filters might also help. TVs in the bedroom generally rob you of sleep. If you need to watch TV before bed, don't watch things that will excite you mentally or emotionally. Set the timer to turn the TV off if you regularly fall asleep while watching shows before bed.

6: Managing the Downside of Shift Work

Shift work is hard on the body, creating cardiovascular, digestive, and sleep issues. Shift work is considered to be any work outside of a steady nine-to-five work schedule. However, those working night shifts are hit by the worst health concerns. Many people doing shift work notice a decrease in quality of life and a general feeling of being unwell. Night-shift workers generally have poor-quality sleep and sleep less than people who work regular hours, thus accumulating sleep debt.[13]

- If you work long shift hours and are allowed by your employer to take a short nap, try to take a mini nap (twenty minutes) once or twice during the shift.[14]
- Keep the same eating schedule on your days off. On the days you work, eat every three to four hours and have your warm meals at work, if possible.
- Don't drive if you are sleepy. In this situation, taking a short nap before driving will help save lives.
- Keep the same sleep schedule on the weekends or days off and adjust your sleep schedule a day or two before the start of your next shift to prevent drowsiness while you work.
- Sleeping in the day can be a little more challenging than at night, but with a little preparation, it's doable. Make sure that family and friends are aware of and respectful of your sleep hours and needs. Ensure you have a comfortable and quiet place to sleep during the day. Silence any distractions as best you can. Foam earplugs and eye masks may improve your sleep.
- Try your best to catch up with your sleep debt. Get in extra sleep hours whenever you can. The more sleep loss we have, the less capable we are of recognizing it. Waiting too long to catch up on your sleep deficit won't do you any good. As sleep debt mounts, its health consequences increase.
- Try to manage your stress effectively and eat a balanced and healthy diet to help ameliorate the harmful effects of shift work.
- For people doing night shifts, taking a ninety-minute nap before going to work seems to help with alertness and memory tasks.[15]

7: Take Back Your Bedroom

The bedroom should be a place you can relax and unwind.

- Don't bring your work into your bedroom. Remove all the clutter and things like calendars and to-do lists that will keep your mind engaged.
- Paint your room in the green, blue, or brown hues to make yourself more calm and grounded. Go with the color that relaxes you even if it's something unusual. It is your bedroom, your sanctuary.
- Place a few drops of essential oils like clary sage, chamomile, or lavender on your pillow to create mild aromatherapy to relax you.
- Choose a comfortable mattress; it should not be too soft or too hard. Creating proper lumbar support will help you stay comfortable and provide better sleep.
- The bed should be used primarily for sleeping and having sex. No eating in bed. No working in bed. No kids and pets in bed overnight.

- If you cannot sleep, then get up and do something else while keeping the lights low. Avoid surfing the net or checking social media. Instead, do something relaxing. Read a book, do a puzzle, meditate, or listen to soft music. If your mind is too active thinking of all the things that need to be done, write them down somewhere and take slow, deep breaths. Watching your breath will help to calm you down.
- Wake up to an alarm clock that gradually gets louder or has a soothing tone. Once your sleep patterns are established, you most likely won't need an alarm clock.
- If you are a particularly anxious and tense individual, progressive muscle relaxation is a wonderful tool for bringing on the relaxation response to help you sleep better. Starting at the feet and moving up to your head (or, if you prefer, go the other way), progressively tighten major muscle groups for five to ten seconds as you take a slow, deep breath. Then release and relax the muscle as you slowly breathe out. Move on to the next muscle group when you feel ready. Paying attention to the difference in feeling between a tense muscle and a loose muscle is important. Take care not to hurt yourself by applying intense pressure. Apply enough pressure to feel the tension. You will get better with practice. For example, starting on one side of your lower body, for your foot, curl your toes downward; for your lower leg, tighten your calf muscle by pulling your toes toward you; and for your upper thigh, squeeze your thigh muscles. Repeat on the other side of your body. For the upper body, starting with your hand, clench your fist. For the entire arm, tighten your biceps by pulling your forearm toward you while clenching your fist. Do the same on the other side of your body. For the torso, starting with your buttocks, tighten them by pulling your buttocks together. For the stomach, suck your belly button in, and for the chest, tighten by taking a deep breath. Lastly, moving up to the neck and shoulders, raise your shoulders up to touch your ears and hold it. Open your mouth wide enough to stretch your jaw, and then scrunch your eyelids tightly shut.[16,17]
- Do a body scan to identify trouble areas. Following the same pattern as progressive muscle relaxation, move through major areas of your body and sense how they feel. Spend a few seconds and observe for any sensations of heat or cold, pain or numbness, tightness or heaviness, or any other sensation. Once you can identify the sensation, take a deep breath. Imagine the breath is a white or yellow glowing light moving from your belly toward the trouble area and healing it as you exhale. If you don't feel any sensation during your scan, move on to the next area, all the while being aware of and keeping your breath

steady. You can do a scan of your body before practicing progressive muscle relaxation or try it by itself as a relaxation tool.

8: Regular Exercise Can Help You Sleep Better

Exercise has shown to have a lot of benefits overall, including sleep benefits.[18] Cardiovascular exercises are more stimulating than resistance exercises and should not be done close to bed. Working out four to eight hours before bed seems to help people fall asleep quicker and have a deeper, better quality of sleep.[19]

9: Epsom Salt to the Rescue

Some people find that taking a warm Epsom salt bath is helpful for enhancing sleep. The Epsom salt, along with the warm water, helps relax tense muscles, which aids in having a relaxing sleep after the bath. Use one to two cups of Epsom salt and keep your baths to forty-five minutes max—twenty minutes seems to be ideal for most people. Keep the water temperature as warm as you can handle, but not too hot. The magnesium sulfate in Epsom salt will pull water out of your body, so stay hydrated. Keep a big bottle of cool water close by and sip throughout the bath. Epsom salt baths may also drop your blood pressure and make your muscles a bit weak, so stand up slowly after the bath. If you are someone who enjoys taking baths, then doing this type of therapeutic bath two to three times a week may help if you have sleep issues.

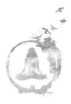

RULES FOR *Exercise*

Exercise is not about going to the gym every day and working out for hours. That is the picture that comes to the mind of most people when they hear the word *exercise*. Exercise means to move beyond our daily activities to improve and maintain good health.

The following are some of the health benefits from exercise:

- More physical endurance, so you can accomplish more in your day
- Better mood
- Improved memory
- A stronger, more efficient heart and lower blood pressure
- A stronger immune system
- Reduced systemic inflammation
- Stronger bones
- An efficient insulin response
- Better stress management
- A more restful, deeper sleep[1,2]

1: The Best Exercise Is the One You Enjoy Doing

There is no rule that says you cannot enjoy exercise. If you enjoy an activity such as hiking, dancing, walking, skating, swimming, or any physical exertion you do that raises your heart rate and elevates your breathing higher than normal, then that is exercise. If you enjoy it, you will do it more regularly, and the whole point of any activity is sustainability and repetition to reap the health benefits. If you can do this activity three times a week for at least half an hour each time, then you are on the right track. Studies have shown that even exercising for as little as five minutes at high intensity is beneficial.[3] The goal here is to make movement a priority. Even less intense exercises such as yoga and tai chi are beneficial, especially if we lead stressful lives. So find something you enjoy and do it regularly.

2: To Stretch or Not to Stretch, That Is the Question

The research on stretching is inconclusive. Furthermore, stretching before exercise does not seem to reduce the risk for injury.[4] If you are concerned with maintaining range of motion for your joints, then stretch after you finish your exercise routine, while your muscles and joints are still warm and pliable. Also, hold the stretch for at least ten seconds[5] and let it gradually release with your own body weight. Do not apply more force. The sensation should be of a dull pressure or pull. There should never be an intense pain when stretching; if there is, you are probably applying too much pressure, or there might be a bigger issue. Stretching regularly will also give you more control over your movements.

- The muscle groups that you use the most may tighten on occasion and make you uncomfortable. Make it a habit to stretch the tight muscles while they are warm.
- Lower back pain is one of the most common complaints and one that can be easily avoided by keeping your core (muscles around your trunk and pelvis) strong. Your workout routine should include exercises that target the core muscles.
- Our spine is a complex and magnificent structure that needs to be protected. Always stabilize your spine and avoid rapid movements under strain. The yoga asanas or poses are a wonderful tool for strengthening and increasing flexibility, especially of the spine. Try to incorporate some form of yoga into your life.

3: The Best Time to Exercise

The time of day you exercise is not as important. If you exercise at night and can sleep like a baby afterward, then go for it. However, if it makes falling asleep difficult, then don't exercise at night. The best time to exercise is when you have the most energy during the day. If losing weight is your goal, then exercising in the morning before breakfast will tap into your fat reserves for energy and help speed up fat loss.

4: Be Accountable to Someone Else

For most people, doing an activity with someone else makes it more fun and keeps you more motivated. Research has shown that being accountable to other people will allow you to exercise for a longer duration.[6] Try to get someone you trust involved in your exercise goals. And if that person has similar health goals as you, then that's a bonus. Both of you can be accountable to each other and can help motivate each other by providing emotional support and encouragement. This in turn provides better self-regulation and self-efficacy.[7] The other option is to hire a coach or recruit someone who has more experience with your health goals to teach you techniques that have worked for them and to keep you accountable and motivated.

5: Don't Weigh Yourself Too Often

Don't use the scale as the only indicator of health. How your clothes fit, how much energy you have in the day, how well you sleep, and how good your mood is are all good indicators that you are benefiting from exercise. Try to weigh yourself just once a week. Our weight can fluctuate throughout the day and on a day-to-day basis. You will get more reliable readings if you pick a time and day of the week and stick to measuring your weight only then.

6: Aerobic v. Resistance Exercise

Doing a mix of aerobic and resistance training is best. Aerobic exercises such as walking, cycling, and swimming strengthen the cardiovascular system, build endurance, and improve memory and attention span.[8,9] Resistance exercises such as yoga, resistance bands, or lifting weights will help strengthen the muscles, and this will improve insulin response, help you gain muscle mass, which will burn more calories, and reduce visceral fat, including fat in the liver.[10,11] How much of each type of exercise you do depends on you. Some days you may gravitate toward cardio—and on another toward resistance-type workouts. Listen to your body; get your clues from it. What is it telling you? Get creative and change things up once in a while. It will keep things interesting and workouts more fun. Our bodies are adaptive and will quickly adjust to any new strain you put on it, so challenge yourself and test your limits, with caution, of course. Give your muscles and joints time to heal after strenuous exercise. Most muscles work with an opposing one (the biceps and triceps in the arm work together, as do the hamstrings and quadriceps in the leg). When we overuse one muscle without working the opposing muscle, that muscle becomes weak, creating an imbalance. Make it a habit to work opposing muscles as well. I would also suggest alternating between upper body and lower body routines to give each muscle group at least forty-eight hours to recuperate.

7: Exercise Outdoors Whenever You Can

If you can have your physical activity outdoors, you will benefit even more. Fresh air, sunlight, and nature are what our bodies need to recharge and rebalance, with the added benefit of cleaner air, vitamin D from sunlight, and the calming effect of greenery. In the winter months, the colder air is denser, with a higher concentration of oxygen, and the cold temperature will make you burn more energy. Whether it's summer or winter, know your own heat and cold tolerance levels. When training outdoors during extreme temperatures, try not to put yourself in danger of hyperthermia or hypothermia.

8: Don't Neglect Proper Nutrition

Nutrition is a big factor in exercise, but not in the way the fitness industry would like you to believe. Our bodies are efficient at conserving essential nutrients, and there is no need to mega-dose yourself on supplements to get the most out of your exercise. If you are looking to add muscle mass, increase your protein consumption by 30 to 50 percent. The timing of protein consumption is important. It is recommended that you eat your protein source within the first two hours after exercise.[12] Supplements like creatine and branched-chain amino acids (BCAAs) help with muscle performance and recuperation for those who are training and need the extra help.[13,14] If you have a balanced diet filled with a variety of fruits, vegetables, good protein sources, good fats, enough fiber, and an adequate amount of water, then you are providing all the nutrients your body needs. If your diet is poor, I would suggest you improve that before you embark on an exercise routine to build your body. It's like building a house with poor-quality bricks and cement; it may look good on the outside, but it won't stand the strong winds.

9: Sit Less, Stand More

Something phenomenal has been happening in society since the dawn of the Information Age. In Western society, we have for the most part become knowledge workers instead of manual laborers. What this means is that people are sitting more than ever at work and have become sedentary. The term "sitting disease" has been coined by the scientific community. Even at home, people spend many hours sitting, glued to the screens in front of their faces. All this sitting is not helpful for your health. Too much sitting is being declared as the new smoking when it comes to its health-risk profile. It can be as damaging to your body as smoking. Being sedentary has been associated with increased risk for cardiovascular disease and diabetes.[15] Furthermore, meeting your exercise requirements, although beneficial, does not negate the ill effects of sitting too much.[16] Granted, this does not paint a pretty picture for most of us, who have to sit for work or while commuting and during leisure activities. What can you do to combat a sedentary lifestyle? Start by being aware of how much you sit and aim to increase your body's movement gradually over time by doing the following:

- Get up at least once an hour, walk around, and do some light stretches. Put an alarm on your phone to remind you.
- Whenever given an opportunity to sit or stand, choose to stand more often.
- Make movement a priority; for example, use stairs instead of the elevator or walk short distances instead of hopping in the car.

- Try to sit less than eight hours per day, because most ill health effects start to materialize beyond this timeline.[17]
- All the movement in the day adds up, so keep moving, and your body will thank you for it.

10: A Few Key Points to Remember

Have a plan and visualize your outcome. What do you want to achieve with exercise? Do you want to have more energy and a better mood, strengthen your bones, raise your good cholesterol, get fit, or fit into that wedding dress? Our minds are powerful machines. Whatever your health goal, breaking it down into smaller, more achievable steps and visualizing the end result will help you achieve it more quickly compared to those who do not have a plan or don't use visualization as part of their process. Break your main goal into smaller, more achievable steps, and set timelines to accomplish them. Be flexible with the timelines and your progress. You will have good days and bad days, which is part of life. Use this to your advantage. On the days when you have more energy, get in a good workout; and when you are feeling down, don't push yourself; relax and recharge. Don't be upset with yourself if you don't achieve your goals within a set time frame, as long as you are progressing in the right direction. Maybe reassess and identify where you could improve to see better results. Did you overlook something important, such as getting enough sleep every day to keep your hunger pangs down, or did you eat more than your share of junk food the past few weeks? Keeping a journal or using a phone app can help track activities and food intake, which can be a tremendous aid when we have a million things to do every day and can't keep track of them all. The benefits of exercise build with time; have patience, take it one day at a time, and watch the magic happen.

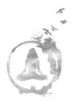

RULES FOR *Stress Management*

When we think of stress, a man or woman clutching his or her head in desperation comes to mind. That is the epitome of what stress may do to us, so we should lower our stress before reaching this state. But all stress is not bad and some stress may actually be useful, depending on the situation. Stress is a normal physiological response.

Classically, the stress response is explained as the fight-or-flight response, where a person confronted by a wild animal will choose to fight or flee the situation. In either case, the body would immediately release the stress hormone adrenaline to increase the heart rate and raise blood glucose to give the individual a quick burst of energy to fight or flee. This situation would normally last a short time, after which the stress hormones would go back to normal and the body would relax and go into a regenerative phase. Fast-forward to the present age; although hopefully no more wild animals are attacking us, our day-to-day lives are becoming more hectic and more demanding than ever. This constant feeling of mental and emotional anguish keeps our stress hormones, particularly cortisol, consistently elevated. Without your body having a chance to relax and revitalize, ill effects start to accumulate. Long-term elevated stress levels may lead to recurrent headaches[1] and increase susceptibility to respiratory infections,[2] chronic pain,[3] fatigue,[4] irritable bowel syndrome,[5] sexual dysfunction,[6] and major depression.[7]

There are two ways to deal with stress. Either remove the stressor or adapt to the stress. In today's world, avoiding stress is nearly impossible. The more practical choice would be to learn to embrace it and manage it well. Let's go through the most common types of stressors people experience and how to best deal with them from a holistic perspective.

1: Physical Stress

Physical stress is any biochemical stress your body experiences. This may be due to the environment you live in or your lifestyle and diet, which may be causing material damage to your body. The environment we live in includes the air we breathe, the water we drink, the food we eat, the things we put on our bodies, and the radiation we are exposed to. Since World War II, thousands of new chemicals have been invented, a fraction of which have been tested for human safety. Most of these chemicals are toxic to humans. Most of them are also carcinogenic[8,9] and lead to cancer through short- or long-term exposure. How are we supposed to protect ourselves when we don't even know what most of these chemicals will do to us? The simple answer is by being vigilant. Don't blindly trust that whatever products you buy are safe. Read product labels, and if there are a bunch of chemicals that you cannot even pronounce, don't put the product on or in your body. The best solution is not to buy such products at all. If many people refuse such highly synthesized chemical products, then the industry will listen and give us what we want. Implement the following:

- In the house, use nontoxic cleaners such as baking soda, lemon, white vinegar, castile soap, and borax. They have tons of uses; google them and be amazed at how good they can be. If you must, reserve the toxic cleaners for the really tough jobs, although natural cleaners can do a good job on those as well. When used regularly, they will work efficiently and be safer for you.
- There is only so much we can do to minimize our exposure to environmental toxins, but whatever little you do is better than doing nothing at all. We also need to help our bodies' elimination systems remove any absorbed toxins properly. Follow my suggestions in the air, water, food, sleep, and exercise sections as best you can to help to both minimize exposure to toxins and provide optimum support and energy for your elimination systems.
- Herbs like milk thistle, dandelion, and turmeric will help heal your liver and help it detox efficiently. I believe now more than ever we need to help our overburdened bodies with detoxifying efficiently. That is why I have dedicated a whole chapter to detoxification.
- We are also constantly being exposed to an invisible toxin, a.k.a. electromagnetic radiation (EMR). The research is new and hence inconclusive as to its long-term effects,[10] but I would err on the side of caution. When tobacco cigarettes were first mass produced, they were thought to be safe. A quick search online will show you ad campaigns from seventy years ago depicting images of doctors and pregnant mothers smoking. After a few decades of cigarette exposure, we realized how harmful they can be. More and more people are using electromagnetic gadgets with longer exposure times. Our smartphones are on us most of the time, and they constantly emit EMR.

These simple, effective practices can help you minimize exposure to EMR:

- The most effective solution is not to carry these devices on your body or close to your genitals; instead, keep them in your purse or bag.

- When using your wireless phone for a prolonged time, keep it away from your head by using the speakerphone function or a wired headset.
- When you sleep, put your cell phone away from your body, out of reach, or keep it in airplane mode if you need it next to you. The same precautions go for most electronics that emit EMR (laptops, tablets, radios, etc.).
- Please don't give children cell phones to use. Their growing bodies and thinner skulls can absorb two to ten times as much radiation as adults'.[11,12] If their safety is an issue, give them an emergency cell phone to use to minimize radiation exposure.

2: Mental and Emotional Stress

There is no shortage of stress in this world. From the moment you wake up to the time you go to sleep, you likely have to deal with mental and emotional stress from all areas of life. There could be stress from your parents or siblings. You might be a caretaker for your parents, and your siblings are not helping out. This could lead to burnout and adrenal exhaustion, which is when your adrenals, your stress glands, cannot manage the cortisol output you require. There could be stress about work. You might not be acknowledged for the hard work you put in, and you might have been passed over for the promotion or raise you were promised. This could make you depressed and lead you to unhealthy coping behaviors, such as eating junk food, smoking, or drinking. You might not get along with a coworker, and every time you see her it infuriates you, which could raise your heart rate and blood pressure. The list of life's stressors can be endless.

Social media can be a huge contributor to our stress as well. One of the reasons is the addictive factor of constantly needing to check different platforms and getting anxious when you cannot. The other, even bigger, issue is the way people perceive their life compared to others on social media. Let me explain; most people post only positive instances in their lives, and this can create an imbalanced view of their real lives. When you look at all your friends' lives online, you may feel inadequate or unhappy with your own life. You might think your friends are having a better life than you because they never reveal any of their hardships. What can you do if you are experiencing these feelings? Realize that everyone goes through hardships and that what you see online may not be the complete picture. If checking social media is disrupting your life and creating anxiety and stress, then consider removing the apps from your smartphone or any other devices you check and only check them using a browser where you need to log in each time. This may reduce the frequency of your interaction and lessen some of the associated stress.

Another key contributor to our stress is the news we are exposed to regularly. The media has a way of creating fear and stress in us by what they report. Notice how you feel when you watch the news. Does your body tense up? Do you get anxious, and does your breathing get fast and shallow? Is your mind occupied throughout the day by what was on the news? If you notice these things, then you have found a major trigger for stress in your life. Instead of absorbing unsolicited news, read or watch what interests you and minimize exposure to negative news.

In a perfect world, everyone would live in harmony and there would be no war or famine, no rat race to survive, no greed for power. Unfortunately, that reality is not on the horizon just yet. In the meantime, in the real world, we have to deal with all the challenges that life throws at us. Our minds are constantly churning out thoughts like a factory. And thoughts lead to emotions. Some thoughts generate stronger emotions than others. If you experience undesirable thoughts on a regular basis, they can spiral down a negative path if left unchecked and lead to feelings of helplessness, anxiety, and depression. One of the most important things we can do is monitor our day-to-day mental activity. The beauty of observing your thoughts is that the more you look at them, the less frequent they become, just like smoke disappearing as you look at it. Tools such as breathing and meditation techniques are invaluable resources for learning to control your thoughts and managing stress. Use them regularly and reap the benefits.

3: Breathing Techniques

Your breathing is the only vital body function that is both voluntary and involuntary, meaning that you can control your breathing, and if you let go, your body will take over. Because of this connection, controlling your breath is a direct path into controlling your mind. Slowing down your breathing is one of the best ways to overcome the stress response. Breathing correctly is the first step. Most of us are chest breathers, as discussed earlier. This is a shallow way of breathing that gives us little oxygen and makes us breathe faster. Instead of breathing vertically, we need to breathe horizontally through abdominal or belly breathing. This method will entirely fill your lungs with air. As you inhale, your belly should rise, and as you exhale, it should fall naturally (refer to "Rules for Air," rule 11). As you do this type of breathing over time, you will notice naturally being less stressed and more resilient.

Yoga teaches several other breathing techniques that are worth learning about. Alternate nostril breathing is my favorite. I teach it often to my patients who have a hard time quietening their minds. The basic concept of this breathing technique is to balance the hemispheres of the brain by alternating the breaths taken through the nostrils. The way it works is that you block your left nostril with a finger and breathe in through the right, then block the right nostril with another finger and breathe out through the left. Without removing your finger, breathe back in through the left nostril, and then cover it and breathe out through the right. This completes one cycle. You would continue by breathing back in through the right nostril and doing the whole process again several times until you feel a sense of calm and reduction in anxiety levels. Don't breathe fast while doing this; follow your natural breathing rate or slow it down a bit, and don't use this technique when one or both of your nostrils are blocked; you will only hurt yourself.

Another great stress-management strategy to consider taking on is tai chi or qigong. These are ancient practices that employ a form of movement meditation along with controlled breathing designed to bring on improved health by harnessing the power of the qi (pronounced *chi*), or energy within us.

4: Meditation, the Bridge to Your Salvation

If untrained, our minds for the most part will jump from thought to thought like a monkey. Meditation is like exercise for the brain, but it is even more than that. It has a profound influence on our mood and physical health as well, from reduction in stress,[13] anxiety,[14] depression,[15] and inflammation,[16] to improved sleep[17] and decrease in chronic pain.[18] Everyone is getting on the meditation bandwagon. Top executives and high-powered people are embracing this technique and seeing wonderful results.

When people think of meditation, they may think of monks sitting silently for hours, and this deters most of us from trying meditation. Starting with just five minutes every day and building up from there is all you need. However, just like anything worth doing, the benefits start appearing through regular practice. There is no one perfect meditation. The best meditation is the one that works for you at where you are in your life. This may change as you evolve mentally and spiritually. The goal with any kind of meditation is to go with the flow and not to resist. You are trying to be still and quiet within yourself, no matter how hectic life gets around you. With time and practice, it will become easier, and research is showing that experienced meditators are showing actual changes in the form and function of their brains with improved cognitive and emotional parameters.[19]

Meditation has become so profuse and dynamic that several subspecialties have developed. However, it all boils down to two main forms of practice: focused meditation and mindfulness-based meditation. With the first, you focus on a single object, most commonly your breath or a mantra such as "om," considered a universal sound. Visualization also falls under this type of practice. With mindfulness meditation, the objective is to observe what is happening inside and outside of you. All manners of perception are fair game. The goal is to be an impartial witness to any experience, doing it without any reservation or judgment and being completely detached. You can start with one perception, such as your thoughts or feelings, and move on to sounds or smells or sensations within your body. Do not react; just monitor the experience. Be the oak tree, allowing the wind to blow through its leaves and the birds to sit on its branches without reacting. In the end, both of these forms of meditative practice are designed to train your mind to a point where you will eventually reach a state of inner silence and a deeper sense of your true being without emotional reactivity, but with calm awareness.

To start the meditative practice, try the most basic form of meditation: observing your breath. You can focus your mind on the sensation of air flowing past the tip of your nose or your belly rising and falling. Whichever sensation you best perceive is the one to choose. If the mind starts to wander, don't get upset; that's the nature of the mind. Just observe that it's wandering off, and gently bring your attention back to your breath. If focusing on your breath is difficult, you can start by using affirmative phrases like "I am strong" or "I am healthy" and visualize these words. If visualizing is difficult, you can chant them. As you can see, there is no right or wrong way; it's bringing it into your way that matters. Most people find it easiest to meditate while sitting with legs crossed. However, you can do it whichever way suits you. Do it standing, walking, sitting, or even lying down, if you can stay awake. You can incorporate meditation into your daily activities. You can walk and pay attention to how your feet touch the ground, and that can be your meditation. You can observe people's eyes or ears in detail, seeing the subtle differences, and that can be your meditation. You can sit and feel the sensations of itching on your body without trying to scratch them, and that could be your meditation. Anything and everything can help you reach closer to the peace of mind you desire. Try different forms of meditation and see what sticks. Practice it regularly and reap the benefits. It's that simple.

Bringing awareness into your thoughts helps break any negative thought patterns. Doing a short meditation before any stressful event in your life, such as before giving a presentation, will help calm your nerves and make you more productive. The objective is consistency; pick a time in the day when you will have five to ten minutes to yourself, and meditate. If it's right before sleep, you will have the added benefit of having a deep, restful sleep. With time, reaching a point where you can dedicate thirty minutes daily for meditative practices is a realistic approach that should be sustainable.

5: Nature to the Rescue

Remember the last time you were in nature. Maybe you went for a walk in the park or hiking through the woods. Imagine that for a short while. How did you feel? Were you at peace? Were you happier? I bet thinking back to those memories made you feel relaxed. It's no coincidence; nature has the power to de-stress you and bring you moments of clarity and peace of mind. Countless studies show the amazing calming and restorative effects of being exposed to nature. Walking in nature just for fifty minutes seems to improve the mood and memory of people with major depressive disorder.[20] Another study showed that compared to urban walking, walking in nature showed reduction in anxiety and improvement in working memory for the participants.[21]

Nature is such an important tool in counterbalancing our stressful lives that it is being supported and used in Japan as a therapeutic mode of stress management. The practice of shinrin-yoku, or "forest bathing," has been in use for some time in Japan. During shinrin-yoku, participants take guided tours in forests, where they engage with and appreciate their surroundings using all their senses. This behavior seems to reduce and normalize blood pressure and improve the immune system of the participants. These health benefits have been attributed to organic compounds, given off by the trees, that the participants would inhale naturally during their walks.[22]

With so many advantages for being exposed to nature, it seems a no-brainer that we all should strive to incorporate this behavior into our stressful lives. Whenever your day gets hectic and your mind is running a mile a minute, try to get out into any park or green space and walk around slowly while appreciating the beauty around you. Preferably, do so without being glued to your smartphone so that all your senses can get their share of nature. As you slow down, notice the nature around you. Maybe you will identify a tree you have never seen before or a flower that takes your breath away. As you walk slowly, your breathing and heart rate will also slow down, bringing your stress levels back to normal. Your mind will put on the brakes in response, and the peace you crave will follow.

6: Use a Purge Journal to Empty Your Mind

This last technique is a simple tool that I use regularly to help my patients manage their stress effectively. Our minds are scary little creatures. We are prone to dwell more on things that could go wrong than things that could go right, and these obsessive negative thoughts can rob us of the happiness and serenity we need. One of the habits of our minds is to keep repeating the same thoughts over and over in an attempt not to forget things. This can be a learned behavior and is taxing on your mental resources, taking time away from constructive thoughts. The beauty with writing down your thoughts is that it gives your mind a physical location for your worrisome thoughts, removing the need for the mind to remember them anymore. This is a great technique for all you worrywarts out there, especially if you are the type that stays up at night pondering and planning, which robs you of precious sleep. All you have to do is to keep a journal next to your bed and, before going to bed, write down things that bothered you that day, mentally and emotionally, or any other thoughts and feelings that occupy your mind. You may also write down planned-out thoughts for the future or to-do lists. You can do this at any point during your day, not just at night. By purging your mind regularly, you will train your mind to not keep ruminating on negative thoughts and focus more on the positive.

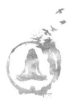

RULES FOR *Relationships*

W e are social beings. We need relationships to grow and evolve as human beings and to survive. Having people or someone in your life you can open up to and be real with has shown to have positive health effects through the comfort of knowing that you will be provided the necessary support during times of need. This type of stress buffering makes you believe that you can cope with adversities more effectively, thus lowering stress levels and preventing undesirable health outcomes.[1] Nowadays, most of us strive to live autonomous, independent lives, and we pride ourselves on our self-sufficiency. But for most of history, and looking at other cultures, having a community network of interdependence has helped humans survive and thrive. I believe there is a benefit for people who put more value in relationships and stronger community networks. It starts with understanding and appreciating all the relationships one develops throughout life and the ways to preserve and improve these relations. There are all kinds of relationships: family, friendships, acquaintances, partnerships, and the list goes on. My suggestions here are by no means specific to every situation, and if any of them upsets you, my apologies.

1: Family Relationships

Familial relations can be the most complex to navigate. They are at the core of our emotional health, since most of us have spent considerable time with family members, especially during our formative years, when we developed our sense of worth and other immutable characteristics. Here are some suggestions:

- Respect your parents, even if they have not been the best parents. You don't have to like them, but they deserve your respect. Remember, no one is taught how to be a parent, and they did their best with the knowledge and abilities they had at that time to raise you. If you are a parent yourself, you will understand.
- Be a friend to your brother or sister. If you already have a strong bond, maintain it. If there are rivalries, get past them. Holding on to anger only hurts one person: you. You don't have to become best friends with your siblings, but holding on to resentment is not healthy. Be the bigger person and extend the olive branch. Blood truly is thicker than

water. You never know when and how they may surprise you with their love, generosity, and affection.

- Cherish your grandparents if you are fortunate enough to have them present. You are a product of their genes. Get to know them and their history. You may be amazed as to what an incredible fountain of knowledge they can be, and they can help you discover your roots and how things are connected.

- Aunts and uncles and cousins all play a vital role in your familial cohesiveness, so try your best to be on good terms with all of them. You may have an aunt, uncle, or cousin who is as close as a parent or sibling, and then there are relatives who get under your skin. In such situations, don't engage them; just smile and move on.

2: Friendships

Friends are a delightful part of our lives because in most cases they are there by choice. Our best friends are our best friends for a reason. They satisfy a need that no amount of money can buy. You both saw in each other a quality you liked and admired, and it brought you closer and created a bond that would last as long as you choose. Best friends are like family, sometimes even closer. Don't take this relationship for granted. Cherish it. Ideally, it's a mutually symbiotic relationship where both people are equal and trust and care for each other. If trust is broken, mend it quickly. Be honest with each other. Being able to share your thoughts and feelings and getting honest feedback from someone you trust may help you form better judgments in life and, as a consequence, improve your odds of surviving and thriving. Throughout your life, people may emerge to guide, support, or motivate you. Some may stay and become lifelong friends, and some may leave. Sometimes friendships are not meant to last forever, and trying to hold on to one that is not viable is not healthy.

If you are shy, know that it's not the quantity of friends you have but the quality of your friendships. An easy way to find or make friends is by doing things you enjoy and being yourself around people. If you like pottery or ballroom dancing, for example, join a class teaching these things and connect with someone there. Being open to the possibility of forming friendships is the first step, and no matter where you are, you increase the odds of making a friend.

3: Acquaintances

The people we see occasionally also need to be acknowledged. These relationships have the potential to become good friendships, so maintaining a good association with all the people you meet is the best way to go. In general, treat people how you want to be treated. Every encounter with another human being teaches us valuable life lessons.

4: The Law of Cause and Effect Is Real

How you treat others will come back to you in some shape or form. Some call this karma. A while back, I was on the bus going to university when someone got on and didn't have enough money for the fare. He was asking around for help, and when he came to me, I gave him five dollars to cover his ticket. He was so thankful. I told him to pay it forward and left it at that. That day in school, when I went to buy a textbook, the cashier gave me a huge discount to my surprise and told me that the book was recently marked down in their system but was not yet updated on the price tag. I don't know if this was just a coincidence or karma, but I was very happy to save that money, and I felt it happened because I helped that individual on the bus. I believe the intentions behind our actions are just as important as our deeds. When I helped that man on the bus, I genuinely wanted to help him, with no expectations of reciprocity or future reward, and I think that is why I was rewarded.

An important consequence of good deeds is the happiness they can bring. Positive health, happiness, and longevity have been associated with kindly emotions and helping behaviors, so long as you don't get overwhelmed by helping others.[2] When you do good or bad deeds for someone, the universe reciprocates. The lesson here is to be more compassionate with your fellow human beings and treat everyone you meet with respect and dignity no matter their social or economic position in life.

5: Don't Make Promises You Know You Cannot Keep

Keep your word, always. It's the most important part of any relationship. Only death or extreme sickness is a good excuse for breaking your word. Knowing this, don't make empty promises you know you won't be able to keep. This resonates deeply with me because of a childhood experience I will never forget. When I was around fourteen years old, one day in school, during gym class, I was not feeling well and was sitting out of the day's activities. Some of my classmates had left their watches with me for safekeeping. I must have been distracted and misplaced one of the watches without realizing it. The classmate whose watch I lost was punished by his parents, and I was called in to the principal's office and reprimanded. I didn't mind being lectured to, but I felt terrible for my classmate for having to go through this ordeal. I believe I gave him my watch in restitution, but ever since then I have vowed to always keep my word.

6: Honesty Is the Best Policy

When I observe small children, I find their brutal honesty to be innocent and refreshing. Somewhere along the line, our ego develops and we start telling small lies to protect it. Unchecked, it can spiral out of control. Usually, once a lie is told, one has to keep lying to cover up the previous lies, and eventually the truth comes out anyway. This is mentally exhausting, and the anxiety that it can cause may have negative health consequences, such as difficulty sleeping and digestive problems. But there is a difference between lying for personal gain and telling a white lie to protect someone else. For example, lying to your boss and taking credit for someone else's work is obviously wrong, but telling your significant other they look skinny in their jeans is acceptable, in my book. As you can see, the line can get blurry and sometimes there is no right answer. Lying can be a learned behavior, and being more aware of your thoughts through meditative practice may help you to break this habit. Some say the world is not built for honest people. How does that resonate with you? However we conduct ourselves, in the end, we have to live within our own consciousness. What is this peace of mind worth to you?

7: How to Deal with Enraged People

When someone is angry, it usually indicates unresolved fear, powerlessness, or frustration with a situation. Men show this frustration as anger because it's more socially acceptable, and women show it with tears for the same reason. This is a generalization and by no means universal. How we express ourselves falls on a continuum, and there is no gender difference, only what has been stereotyped and portrayed within each culture.[3]

When someone lashes out at you in anger, don't engage them. Listen calmly and acknowledge them. Try to see the situation from their perspective and work toward a resolution. The anger should diffuse. Most times the situation escalates when the second person engages and retaliates. However, you can only do so much. If at any point you feel your safety is compromised, take yourself out of the situation and ask for help. Run if you have to.

If you are the type of person who gets enraged easily, then learn to recognize your main triggers and avoid them as best you can. Maybe a particular person or situation can set you off. Look into the underlying cause of your anger. For example, you might be enraged when someone cuts into line at the coffee shop and no one says anything. Why do you think that is? Is it because you feel that you have been following the rules and someone else shouldn't be allowed to break the rules and get away with it? Or is it because no one stood up to the line cutter, including you, and you are angry with yourself for being afraid to speak up?

There are many instances I am sure you can recount where countless lives have been affected because of greed and corruption. Realizing the truth that the world can be unfair and that bad things happen to good people all the time doesn't help, but it can make us understand that we need to pick our battles and reserve our energy for the things that really matter.

Meditation can be a great tool to help you become calmer and more in control when faced with a negative situation. A few years back, I would get agitated easily, and little things could set me off. On the advice of a colleague, I went to a meditation retreat for ten days and practiced Vipassanā meditation. When I returned home and turned on my computer, I got the blue screen of death. Before meditation, I would have become angry, but to my surprise, I did not react at all. I was calm and tried for a couple of hours to restore my computer, and I was successful. It might be worthwhile going to one of these meditation retreats and completely submerging yourself into the world of meditation. Visit dhamma.org to get more information on Vipassanā meditation. They have meditation centers throughout the world and charge nothing for their courses; they are run solely on donations.

8: Your Significant Other

Countless books have been written about romantic relationships, and most of them give great advice; however, it all boils down to one thing: communication. Men and women process information differently. We are essentially different creatures when it comes to behavior within a relationship.[4] To have a harmonious relationship, we need to be aware of how the opposite sex thinks and what they prioritize in their life. This way we can better understand them and learn how we can communicate and interact with each other effectively. It is the quality of your relationship with your significant other that is crucial for health, as it has shown to have positive effects on psychological well-being.[5]

How men and women think and behave is certainly not set in stone. Like anything, it falls on a continuum. There is also gender fluidity, where the relationship dynamics will be unique in each situation. There will be differences and similarities, and sometimes the boundaries get blurred. For the most part, I believe same-sex relations may have an advantage when it comes to communication and understanding each other.

With changing times, some men are adapting and taking on a more nurturing role in relationships, and some women are taking on a more dominant role as breadwinners. This is the new norm in some families. However, there will be certain behaviors that will always remain and irritate your partner. Those are the small issues that will add up, if not resolved, and can lead to bigger problems down the road. Most of my relationship advice comes from a heterosexual viewpoint, through experience-derived knowledge.

Men, for the most part, tend to be direct and tell you what they want. Women tend to be indirect and move around the subject matter. If this is the communication style within the context of your relationship, then know this about each other and learn to recognize it. For women, I would suggest being more direct when talking with your man. If you want him to do something, tell him exactly what you want and when you want it done. Give him a realistic timeline and it will get done; otherwise, it might be a while before he gets to it. Also, most men want to be appreciated for every little thing we do; it feeds our ego and makes us feel needed.

For men, one of the most important things you can do for your significant other is to listen with more care and attention when she talks. She will give you clues and hints for what she needs. If you're watching TV, don't just nod your head while she talks. Pause the show or turn the TV off. Then turn to face her and listen intently to what she is saying. Your woman wants attention from you. She craves it. Give her your attention. It's one of the simplest things you can do to keep her happy. This is not to say that men don't want attention from their significant other. I think spending regular quality time with each other will help.

Most men's main drive in life is to acquire wealth. An attack on their career will create problems. When it comes to processing emotions, men need their space to process their feelings; that's why they have their man caves. Women, on the other hand, need to vocalize their feelings and be heard to process their emotions. Men respond better when serious conversations are held while doing an activity, such as driving or building something. If he doesn't want to talk about something, don't push it. Let him know that you will be there when he is ready to talk.

Women's main drive is to maintain harmonious relationships. If there is an issue in a relationship, women need to talk about it, usually with other women, to figure out how to resolve the issue, or just to be heard to empty themselves. Men normally will not talk to anyone about something bothering them, unless they have someone they are comfortable confiding in.

For resolving conflicts, here are some helpful tips for both sexes:

- Use "I" statements, not "you" statements.
- Don't attack his or her character; you will get nowhere. Instead, tell him or her how the behavior or situation made you feel.
- Never place blame.
- Never create ultimatums.
- Never play the "who was right or wrong" game. Try to remove your ego from the equation.
- Never bring up past issues or arguments; stay on the subject matter.
- If you are in a highly emotional state, then put off the conversation until you have cooled down and can discuss the problem rationally. You can write down your feelings while they are fresh and then assess their validity when you are calmer.
- At a time when both of you are ready, discuss how you feel and try to recognize and respect each other's feelings.

- If your partner has personally hurt you, then use "I" statements to tell him or her how it made you feel. Make sure that when one person is speaking, the other is listening and acknowledging their partner's feelings. For example, "I felt ignored by you when we were with your friends, and it made me feel unloved." The partner can acknowledge this by saying, "I never realized my behavior at the party was bothering you. It was not my intention, and I am sorry for making you feel unloved. It won't happen again, and I do love you." This can be followed by hugging your partner.
- The goal is to come up with a solution together. Don't wait until things get out of hand.

9: Work Relationships

It's not a good idea to mix work and private life. Work relations, for the most part, classify as acquaintances. Office politics can be tricky, and the bigger the organization, the more complex it becomes. I would advise against getting into the office politics of gossip and manipulation. Information is power, so keep yourself informed on who the main players are in your organization, where the power lies, and how you fit in that hierarchy. Try your best to be on good terms with everyone, and avoid or be on good terms with those who have malicious intentions. Most of us can spend quite some time interacting with the people we work with, and some of them can become lifelong friends through the process of sharing our thoughts and feelings.

People can become romantically inclined with coworkers, and sometimes these types of relationships work out and even turn into significant relationships. However, before deciding to become involved with someone you work with, you need to play out different scenarios in your head. What if the relationship doesn't work out? Will it be awkward for both of you at the workplace, or will it be okay? Is he or she your superior or boss, and how will that dynamic work? Work through all the angles. The last thing you want to do is lose your job over this.

If you have people working under you, learn to recognize their strengths and weaknesses. When managing others, learn to delegate tasks responsibly while trying not to micromanage. Give them the opportunity to prove themselves. Everything doesn't have to be perfect. Realize the value of people, not only for what they can do, but for who they are as human beings.

10: Relationship with God and Your Spiritual Self

Studies show that religion or spirituality protects against cardiovascular diseases. Among male African American churchgoers, higher religiosity translated to fewer depressive symptoms.[6,7] If we look at our relationship with God logically, it would seem one-sided, but for many, the belief in a higher power may be therapeutic and worth pursuing. Most believers tend to think of God in times of trouble, but I would suggest making our connection with the omnipresent a more continuous venture.

Regardless of our belief systems, we need to be more caring and kind to each other. This makes us spiritual and connects us all as one. Furthermore, having an attitude of gratitude and generosity brings happiness[8] to those who practice it and seems to be the foundation for creating a more holistic connection with the higher self.

11: Relationship with You

Last is our relationship with ourselves. We know no one better than ourselves, and if you don't, then get to know yourself; it's the most important relationship you will ever have. You are born alone and you die alone, and between those events you have to spend every waking moment with yourself, interspersed with moments of interactivity with others. If you are not comfortable in your own skin, then living a peaceful life will be challenging. Discover yourself, however necessary, through adventure, introspection, learning a new skill, or creating relationships. You must learn what makes you tick and what is important to you.

Realize your limitations and your strengths. Your limitations don't make you weak; they make you human. You can try to improve your weaknesses, but if doing so takes too much energy, it's not worth it. I was not good at calculus in university, and no matter how much I tried, I could not comprehend beyond a certain point. I had to change majors and follow my passion into natural medicine. Once I did, things started to flow more smoothly, and I was able to achieve my goals. Sometimes you are not good at something because it doesn't resonate within your core and give you joy. Instead, focus on your strengths and build on those. We try to be everything, and most times that ends up with us doing nothing. Learn to love and accept yourself with all your perceived flaws, and all your other relationships will reflect back to you what you put into your own relationship with yourself.

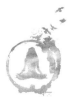

RULES FOR *a Healthy Mind*

Most of this book focuses on a healthy body, but you cannot have a healthy body without a healthy mind, and vice versa. How you think and how you feel will have an impact on your health, period. Remember the last time you felt a strong emotion for a sustained period of time. How did you feel in your body? Did your appetite diminish or increase? Did you sleep well? Did you have pain in your body? Your mind has a strong influence on your health. Similarly, having poor health can influence your mind negatively. Eating highly processed foods regularly can depress your mood and lead to mood swings, while consuming a variety of fruits, vegetables, and omega-3-rich fish has shown to lower the incidence of depressive episodes.[1]

I am not trying to say that we need to always be happy to be healthy. It is unrealistic and may even be counterproductive. As human beings, we are supposed to feel all the emotions our mind generates. There is a purpose and reason for everything that we feel. Your anxiety may propel you to be more cautious. Your anger or fear may propel you to face a situation and take action. A lot of decisions are made based on how we feel about a subject matter. You may fool yourself into thinking that you made a decision based on research and hard facts, but most of the time we go with our gut instinct.

The problem happens when we let our emotions take control of our lives completely and let it become pathological in nature. Sometimes it may not be in our control and life circumstances can send someone down a spiral from which they may not recover, but most of the time one can see the signs and interject in time. Being mentally healthy means being able to bounce back from adversity by developing the ability to cope with difficult situations.

The other aspect of a healthy mind has to do with your mental prowess or cognitive abilities. For some individuals, getting older means a decline in intellectual ability, but it does not have to be so. Certain cognitive abilities, such as evaluating emotions of others and vocabulary, seem to improve with age, and a large-scale study suggested that there may be no age at which humans perform at peak on all mental tasks and that our cognitive abilities change as we age.[2]

Mental health is a complex and powerful topic that is ever evolving. We need to realize its potential in our lives and manage it as best we can through being mindful of our mental processes. A good diet with wholesome food rich in omega-3s, regular exercise, stress management, and high-quality sleep are some of the basics we have already covered, and these are paramount for mental health. But beyond these strategies, let's see what else we can do to keep a healthy mind into our golden years.

1: Good Workouts for Brain Health

We spend a lot of time and effort exercising our muscles, but when it comes to our brain, where are the gyms for a good brain workout? Thinking is the primary exercise for the brain, but the right type of thinking is needed to make new neural connections and strengthen preexisting ones.

- One of the best ways to improve your brain's power is to stop looking for shortcuts to problems and think through solutions the old-fashioned way by doing the grunt work. For example, instead of using the calculator, do the math mentally, or instead of using the GPS, visualize the map in your head. It may take a bit longer, but the side effect is a sharper mind.

- If you want to improve your focus and memory[3] throughout adulthood, then solve mental problems. The simplest way to do so is to do puzzles, such as word puzzles, crosswords, Scrabble, and sudoku.

- Read about things that intrigue you and make you ponder, and watch movies that are thought provoking. Reading and watching such things will help you assimilate new information, which you can integrate and relate to what you already know. This will help challenge your viewpoints and set patterns, making you develop more questions and a curiosity to learn more.

- Expose yourself to new situations, places, and people. Developing a sense of curiosity about the world around you and seeing the world as a wondrous place full of possibilities will stimulate your brain, releasing a flood of chemicals that will solidify the experience in the mind long term.[4] One of the best ways to do this is to forgo routine and find new ways of doing things. For example, if you always take the same route to work, try a different route, or if you always eat or brush your teeth with your dominant hand, try it with your other hand.

- Challenging your brain is a surefire way to keep your mental machinery well oiled. Learn something new; for example, if you are so inclined, take on a musical instrument and learn how to play it. Keep practicing until you are good at it. Another great challenge is to learn a new language and practice it with people who are native to that language. You will not only develop a marketable skill but make social connections, which will inevitably be rewarding.

2: Embrace Your Emotions

Humans are social and emotional beings. When it comes to the mind, it's the number of neural connections that matter. Similarly, having meaningful connections in one's life transforms us into more resilient beings with more flexible minds. Our perception of positive social connections seems to infuse us with positive emotions, and vice versa.[5] Doing so may help us be more compassionate and emotionally balanced as well. So what can you do?

- Don't burn bridges unnecessarily; keep connections with your loved ones. Nurture and cherish them.
- Try to make new friends or, if you are shy, reconnect with an old friend.
- Connect with your social network regularly. Share your ideas, thoughts, and emotions, and listen without judgment when others speak.
- Join a group of like-minded individuals with a shared interest. It could be anything from role playing or hiking to gardening or reading and discussing literature.
- Volunteering your services is a great way to satisfy our innate need to give to others. Helping the community in any way can enrich your life and give you wonderful memories for a lifetime; the opportunities are limitless.

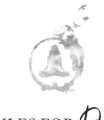

RULES FOR *Detox*

Detox, short for detoxification, is a natural, self-regulatory process of the body. Your main detoxification organs are the liver and kidneys. Your supporting detoxification organs are the lungs, skin, colon, and lymphatic system. They all play pivotal roles in their continuous effort to keep the body healthy and free of toxins. What one needs to realize is that your body is continuously detoxifying day and night without any effort on your part. It's the reason you are still alive. If your liver, for example, didn't do its detoxification job with the toxic buildup of just ammonia, a by-product of protein breakdown, you wouldn't survive more than a few weeks.[1,2] When it comes to detoxification, your main job is to make sure you don't impede the function of these vital organs by continuing to add extra burdens on them.

1: Minimize Assault to Your Detox System

As a starting point, we want to minimize exposing our bodies to unnecessary toxic burdens from unhealthy lifestyle habits. You have probably heard the following countless times, but it's worth mentioning again: avoid or cut back on overconsumption of alcohol, smoking cigarettes, and eating highly processed foods.

Alcoholic liver disease can take years of heavy drinking to develop, but the damage at that point may be irreversible.[3] The beauty of the liver is that it can regenerate itself, and cutting back or refraining from alcohol over time will allow the liver to heal itself and function optimally. To minimize damage to the liver, the CDC recommends that for adults of legal drinking age, men can consume up to two drinks per day, and women can consume one drink per day. They do not recommend averaging this out (in other words, you shouldn't binge drink several drinks in one day and drink less on the other days).[4]

Lighting a cigarette creates more than four thousand harmful chemicals, which will have adverse health effects on almost every organ in the body. Smoking directly damages the lungs, but its toxins can indirectly injure liver cells through the creation of pro-inflammatory cytokines, which over time can lead to liver cancer.[5,6]

Eating chemically processed foods in which the food or drink is made solely from refined ingredients and artificial substances creates an extra burden on our detox system. High fructose levels found within most of these foods can lead to fat deposits within the liver, and over time this can lead to fatty liver disease and insulin resistance.[7]

In addition, if you work with toxic chemicals, such as heavy-duty cleaners and pesticides, use proper protection for your skin, lungs, and eyes by wearing the appropriate barriers on parts of your body that may come in contact with these poisons.

2: Do It Right

The word *detox* has become a fad in the last few years. Celebrities are all doing it, which prompts the public to get intrigued. But if self-directed detox is not done properly, you could possibly harm yourself. For example, some over-the-counter products that claim to help you detox contain strong laxatives. Taking these strong laxatives will flush out your colon, making you feel lighter, especially if you suffer from constipation. However, regular use of such products will make you dependent on them to have a proper bowel movement, without which you could get even worse constipation. I advise caution and prudence when venturing into this territory.

3: Our Toxic World

It's unfortunate, but we live in a toxic world. One cannot escape it. The air we breathe, the water we drink, and the food we eat all have small amounts of harmful substances that our bodies will have to spend extra effort neutralizing and removing. What cannot be dealt with will be stored in our fat cells and connective tissue throughout our bodies for later disposal.

Not burdening our bodies is important, but what is even more important is addressing the root cause and not contributing to the further pollution of our environment. You may think that one person cannot make a difference, but that is not true. What you do will make a difference, and your well-intentioned actions will influence others around you; enough actions will become big enough to make a difference.

4: How to Minimize Your Toxic Impact on the World

Below are some adjustments we can make in our day-to-day lives to reduce our negative impact on the environment:

- Drive cleaner cars, or even better, take public transit if you have access. If you are driving a gasoline car, keep it tuned up. Electric cars are zero emission, and although there was an environmental impact in their creation, their lifetime contribution to pollution can be less than a gasoline car, provided the electricity used to make them came from renewables,[8,9] making them a viable option. Furthermore, some governments are promoting their use by offering considerable rebates, making them more affordable.

- Never flush used car fluids or other waste chemicals from the house into the outside storm drain, which usually runs on the sides of roads. Unlike the sewer drains that go from inside of the house, these storm drains are designed to collect and empty rainwater straight into a water source, and this water is not treated and purified like the water in the sewage system. All hazardous household waste products should be disposed of properly; call your municipality if you don't know where something should go.

- Use nontoxic cleaning products such as baking soda and white vinegar in your day-to-day cleaning. If you need to use a harsher product, make sure to keep the place well ventilated, protect yourself with proper gloves, and don't breathe in the fumes. Furthermore, use nontoxic weed killers on your lawn. Minimizing their use will lessen their environmental impact and also reduce your toxic burden. There are many natural ways to get rid of those pesky eyesores; just do a quick search online. The best, in my opinion, is to pull weeds out from the root by hand or use one of those fancy weed-removing gadgets.

- Plastic bottles and plastic containers are becoming a serious issue. Tons of plastic end up in our oceans in large garbage patches the size of small countries. They get eaten by marine life and end up in our food supply system.[10] Instead of buying bottled water for everyday consumption, use reusable glass or metal bottles and fill them with filtered tap water or regular tap water, if you know it's safe. Keep the plastic bottled water for emergency use. Also, minimize use of plastic bags; instead, use reusable cloth bags for carrying your shopping items. Keep the reusable bags in your car or in a place where you can see them, so that you can take them with you when you go shopping. We are not all perfect, so if you end up using plastic bottles once in a while, don't throw them in the garbage. Recycle them. Many cities have amazing recycling programs, so use them efficiently.

- Any time you buy a new product, realize that there has been an environmental impact in the creation of that product. I am not trying to make you feel bad about buying new stuff, but consider purchasing slightly used or refurbished items whenever possible. You will save money and protect the environment and ultimately yourself by being exposed to fewer toxic by-products. There are some items I would not expect you to buy used, like personal hygiene products, but major things like cars, televisions, and furniture can be bought secondhand in nearly new condition. Also try to minimize the use of disposable and one-time-use products such as Styrofoam cups, plastic plates and utensils, coffee pods, and disposable razors. Instead, opt for their reusable alternatives.

- When renovating your home, adopt eco-friendly methods such as using repurposed or recycled material and more natural plant-based products, such as cork and bamboo.[11] These will release less toxic gas and make living in your home healthier. Plus, their manufacturing and lifetime use will contribute to a lower environmental impact and create more sustainability.

5: Detoxification on a Daily Basis

Now that we have laid the groundwork, let's discuss what you can do on a daily, weekly, and monthly basis to avoid toxins and help your body detoxify itself efficiently.

- Make a conscious decision to avoid things you know to be harmful to your health. For example, keep away from people while they smoke. Inhaling secondhand smoke in an unventilated area is just as bad, if not worse, than smoking yourself.
- When you wake in the morning, the first thing you need to do is drink two to three cups of lukewarm water. If you are not used to drinking that much water all at once, you can start slowly with one cup and gradually build up from there. Add a tablespoon of organic apple cider vinegar to your water to further assist you in your detoxification. This single act alone will greatly help your body get rid of the neutralized toxins your liver and kidney processed the night before.
- Don't sit in your car and idle it for a long time when you first get in. When the engine is cold, the fuel doesn't burn completely, leaving toxic by-products you might inhale. Just idle your car for a minute and drive off slowly until your car warms up.[12]
- If you are like me and have a weak digestive system, taking half a lime or lemon with your meals will make your stomach thank you. This will allow you to break your food properly into smaller pieces to be digested and absorbed. Fewer larger pieces will slip into your bloodstream, preventing immune-system reactions. This is believed to direct more energy toward important body processes such as cellular repair and detoxification.
- Make sure you have regular bowel movements. If you are getting enough fiber in your diet, as we discussed in the food chapter, then that should not be an issue, and the extra water you are drinking will

help the fiber stay soft and easy to pass. Some of the toxins and their metabolites end up in the intestines, and the fiber in your diet will help absorb and mop them up so they don't get reabsorbed back into your blood.[13]

- If you like to use personal-care products on your skin and hair to clean up, beautify, smell good, or moisturize, be aware of the chemicals in those products. Our skin is not as impermeable as we once thought. What you apply on your skin will to some degree end up directly in your bloodstream.[14,15] This mode of chemical delivery is considered worse than consuming it through the digestive system, because it bypasses the liver's main detoxification pathway. When looking at personal-care products, I would avoid getting ones with the following known unsafe chemicals: sodium lauryl sulfate or sodium laureth sulfate, paraben, BHA (butylated hydroxyanisole), BHT (butylated hydroxytoluene), DEA (diethanolamine) and TEOA (triethanolamine), DBP (dibutyl phthalate; pronounced *thal-ate*), DMDM hydantoin, diazolidinyl urea, imidazolidinyl urea, methenamine, quaternium-15, cyclotetrasiloxane and cyclopentasiloxane (also known as D4 and D5), synthetic fragrances, and triclosan.[16] We have come a long way. Now we have options. Alternative chemical-free or chemically reduced products are out there for your consumption. Personally, I have been using a facial moisturizer from Sukin for years, and I love it. Supporting companies that produce green or organic products will funnel more money into research and development of healthier solutions and ultimately give you improved choices in the future.

- We have discussed water consumption, but I cannot emphasize it enough. Make H_2O your friend. You can detox much more efficiently when you are properly hydrated. I would also suggest incorporating a daily gentle detox tea to end your day. My favorite is a detox tea made by Traditional Medicinals; it has a light taste that I enjoy. On a side note, I am not paid by any of the brands that I recommend; they are purely from experience.

- A few times a day, find fresh air wherever possible and take a few fast, shallow breaths followed by a few slow, deep breaths. This will help clear out toxins trapped in your lungs and introduce fresh, oxygenated air. Breathe in and out through your nose only. However, if your nose is blocked, don't force air through it; breathe through your mouth. Some folks may get lightheaded initially from doing this, so do it sitting down if that is the case.

- Using your hands, do a daily dry rub on your body to activate your lymphatic system, which lies mainly just below your skin. Rub your arms and legs in long, even, gentle strokes toward your heart. This will move the lymph within your lymphatic system toward their respective nodes for filtration. Do this before taking a shower, while your skin is dry, as it helps create enough friction. Making it a part of your shower routine will help you to remember to do it. Some folks take it a step further and use a stiff bristle brush with a long handle and brush the skin to exfoliate and create healthier skin.

6: Detoxification on a Weekly Basis

Now that we have seen what we can do on a daily basis, let's discuss strategies to help you detoxify on a weekly basis.

- Eat less red meat, particularly commercially produced cow and pig meat, especially when it's made into other products such as hot dogs, sausages, and deli meats through chemical processing using artificial ingredients. If you can obtain your meat from a humane, organically grown animal source that has gone through only mechanical processing of cutting and mixing solid ingredients, then consuming such meat in a responsible and modest way should not pose a problem. Although poultry and seafood are better choices, they are not necessarily a safer alternative, and we need to do our due diligence when buying them, making sure we know the origin of such meat. As for poultry, typically free range or organic is a better choice, and most wild seafood is a better option than farmed, especially if you are not aware of the farming conditions of the fish you are eating.

- In general, consuming a varied diet of fruits, vegetables, and herbs is the best way to promote a healthier gut and an efficient detox system. Some foods can enhance your detoxification ability and are hepatoprotective in that they protect the liver from damage by toxins, through their antioxidant and anti-inflammatory properties. By strengthening the liver, they allow it to function optimally. Some of them improve the function of the kidneys at removing waste products, through increased urine output. Incorporate the following foods into your diet to improve your detoxification ability:

  » Dandelions:[17,18,19] Eat these raw in a salad, sauté them, or make them in soup. You can eat every part of the dandelion – leaves, flowers, stems and roots. Most people consider these weeds, but now you can think of them as free, highly nutritious liver-helping food. If your lawn is not chemically treated, then just grab these right out of your backyard.

  » Milk thistle:[20,21] Get the seed extract as a supplement. Use this especially if you have regular alcohol consumption or have suffered from viral hepatitis.

- » Turmeric:[22,23] I find it best to use turmeric as a spice in cooking, always making sure to add pepper as well. You can find its extract forms in capsules, but they can get expensive.
- » Garlic and ginger:[24,25] Like turmeric, use these while preparing your food. Make sure to always crush the garlic to activate its sulfur compounds.
- » Parsley:[26] I like to eat this raw as a salad with meals, but you can choose to juice it as well.
- » Globe artichoke:[27] You can eat this however you like; I prefer to eat it pickled.
- » Beetroot:[28,29] You can have this pickled as well or boil it in a pressure cooker and drink the water it was boiled in; then eat the beets as a side dish.
- » Asparagus:[30,31] There are many ways to eat asparagus, but I would say lightly sautéed or roasted is best.
- » Lemon:[32] Have the juice as a refreshing drink or squeeze it on your food. Do not add too much sugar in your juice; try honey instead.
- Eating your meals in a calm, relaxing environment is important for proper digestion and absorption. Being consistently stressed, especially during meals, will raise cortisol levels, which will impede digestion and make the gut lining more porous, and this can lead to intestinal hyperpermeability and a host of unpleasant symptoms.[33] Your body's energies will be wasted by your immune system and less will go toward detoxification.

7: Detoxification on a Monthly Basis

Fasting seems to have gotten a bad reputation, even among some complementary and alternative medicine (CAM) practitioners, because of misinformation and ignorance, but I would like to assure you, when done properly, it is one of the best things you can do for your health. Fasting is one of the most powerful ways to detox efficiently. It is unpleasant and challenging at times, but it is worth it in the long run. A lot of energy and resources are used by the body to digest food, and when we fast, we direct all that energy to restore and renew our cells and organs and clean house.

Technically, a fast should include no food of any sort, just plain water. However, this may be hard for most people, myself included. I generally fast for thirty-six hours, starting from Saturday night to Monday morning, but you can do any variation as long as it's sustained for at least sixteen hours. Most of my patients prefer the weekend fast as well, since they can relax without worrying about work performance. I find it easier to not eat anything. Instead, just drink some herbal teas. If I start to get intense hunger pangs, I eat a few nuts. You may opt to start with a juice fast for the first few times until your body gets used to it. It is important to make sure you get enough fiber the few days before a fast to keep your bowels regular so you don't get constipated after your fast. Eating plenty of fruits and vegetables will take care of that. Break the fast with a light meal of fruits or nuts to avoid shocking your digestive system. Soaking the nuts overnight will make them easier to digest. When you fast, you are removing toxins at an accelerated rate, so any unpleasant symptoms may be heightened. You may get headaches, nausea, diarrhea, constipation, skin breakouts, low energy, and irritability. If these symptoms are really bothering you, break your fast by eating something and you will start to feel better. You may attempt to fast again on another day. Also, try to get as much fresh air and sunlight during your fasts as you can.

Choose to have your fast on a day you know you can relax and not be disturbed. This is not only a time to slow down physically, but mentally and emotionally as well. As your body fasts, you may notice old emotions and negative thought patterns emerging. This is your mind cleaning house as well. Do not resist anything you experience. Just be an impartial observer and let the thoughts and emotions flow through and dissipate. This is a good time for introspection as well. Try to meditate on problems or issues you may be facing, and you may be astonished by how creative your mind can be at finding solutions.

Another great aid to fasting is raw, unfiltered, unpasteurized organic apple cider vinegar, which will have a similar effect to lemon or lime, although more on the detoxifying side. I like Bragg's organic apple cider vinegar. If you don't like the taste of lime or lemon, then this is another option. Consider using it as part of your detoxing protocol. Start with one teaspoon in a cup of water and increase to your tolerance level. Although the vinegar or lemon juice is acidic, the effect will be to make your body more basic. If you suffer from stomach ulcers, don't drink these drinks until your stomach heals. While using this drink, you may feel terrible for the first few fasts, because your body is flushing toxins into your bloodstream faster than your liver and kidneys can process them. Furthermore, you will be changing your gut microbiome by killing off unwanted bacteria, fungi, and parasites. If you find this unpleasant feeling intolerable, then don't use apple cider vinegar during fasts; instead use it as a digestive aid during your non-fast days.

I would advise caution if you suffer from chronic kidney or liver disease, are diabetic, or have active gallstones and gallbladder disease. In such cases, avoid fasts longer than a day and always do them under medical supervision.

Health is a journey, not a destination. There will be ups and downs. Some days you will feel wonderful on a fast, and some days you will feel like crap. That is normal. Take it slowly, and let your intelligent body take care of the rest.

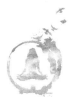

RULES FOR *Cancer Prevention*

Cancer is such a powerful six-letter word that for some it strikes fear in their hearts like nothing else can. I would like to dispel some myths about this stigmatized disease and provide hope. I don't want to belittle anyone who is suffering from cancer of any sort, and if you have been diagnosed with cancer already, please follow the advice of your doctor. The information provided here is strictly preventative, not a cure.

Most people are unaware that everyone has some form of cancer cells in them already. As a result of genetic mutation, for whatever reason, some cells don't die and begin to multiply. It is the job of our immune system to identify such cells and destroy them. Luckily, most times they do an efficient job. It is when these damaged cells begin to grow uncontrollably that they pose a problem and get identified as cancerous and a danger to our health. Cancer has affected humans for centuries, and it seems to be more prevalent now, but our modern lifestyle cannot be entirely to blame. People live longer these days, so there are more chances of genetic mutations with time, and we have more advanced detection technologies now to detect cancers sooner. However, there does seem to be a link between the invention of thousands of new chemical products and the rise in cancer rates.[1,2] The majority of these chemicals have not been tested for long-term safety. These chemicals are being used by us in our day-to-day living, hiding in plain sight in the products we use regularly.

Two interesting theories are beginning to hold some ground in research:

The first theory is the metabolic theory, which states that cancer is caused by a malfunction in the energy production of the cell.[3] The mitochondria are responsible for most of the energy production in our cells, through an oxidative process. This is the primary reason we breathe in air, to absorb oxygen for this process. It appears that there is a drastically reduced number of mitochondria in cancer cells. If this cellular machinery is damaged, the cells have no choice but to resort to the less-efficient fermentation process for energy production. As this happens, the cells need to consume larger amounts of glucose (sugar) to survive by using this inefficient method.[4]

The other theory is that cancer is a reexpression of an ancient preprogrammed trait that has lain dormant. In ancient times, when the earth was more acidic and contained less oxygen, cells used to benefit from being immortal;

they could proliferate unchecked, but as conditions improved, multicellular organisms developed with higher functionality, and immortality was assigned to the sperm and the egg. Now when faced with environmental threats such as unhealthy lifestyle factors that lead to higher acidic states from excess sugar consumption and lower oxygen saturation from inactivity, the cells are reverting to their preprogrammed fail-safe mode and beginning to proliferate ruthlessly in an attempt to survive.[5,6]

Knowing this, let's look at what we can do to minimize the chance of developing cancer.

1: Oxygen and Cancer

It seems that oxygen and cancerous cells don't get along, and it has been theorized that for some cancer cells, such as breast cancer cells, increasing oxygen supply to tissues reduces cancer proliferation, as seen in animal studies.[7] Although still preliminary, there is merit in this theory. A good way to increase the oxygen concentration in your cells is by breathing deeper and using your entire lung capacity. By now, you must be an expert in deep belly breathing, and you now have one more reason to practice it regularly by making it your primary mode of breathing. In my opinion, going for a nice, long, semi-fast walk in nature during the late morning hours is the best time to maximize your oxygen intake. At home, regularly open the windows to let in fresh air and have houseplants, such as peace lily and spider plants. Also, don't burn too many candles, especially during the winter, when the house can have less flow of fresh air. Our red blood cells use iron to bind and transport oxygen from the lungs to the rest of our body. If you are anemic because of low iron levels, eat foods rich in iron. These foods include animal meats and organ meats, especially the liver, as well as sesame seed butter, beans, lentils, dark leafy greens (including seaweed), sun-dried tomatoes, eggs, dried apricots, and peaches.[8]

2: The Benefits of the Sunshine Vitamin

Out of all the vitamins, D_3 seems to have the most research supporting its anticancer properties. It has been shown to reduce the occurrence of many types of cancers, including colon, breast, ovarian, renal, pancreatic, and prostate.[9] This amazing vitamin is made naturally by our bodies in the presence of sunlight. Nearly half of the world population is deficient in vitamin D. Low levels of vitamin D are becoming a global problem in all age groups, even in countries with sun exposure throughout the year. Girls and women in the Middle East seem to have very low levels because of less exposure to sunlight.[10,11] The best source of vitamin D is sunlight. Getting ten to fifteen minutes of direct sunlight on the bare skin of your face, arms, and legs a few times a week is enough to produce the required amount of vitamin D. The more skin surface area exposed to sunlight, the more vitamin D you will produce. If you are darker skinned or older, you will need more time to produce enough vitamin D. The sunlight ultraviolet (UV) index needs to be above 3 to make vitamin D. This usually happens between 10 a.m. and 3 p.m. If your shadow is longer than you are when you stand in the sun, then you may not be making enough vitamin D. Many people in the northern hemisphere are deficient in vitamin D because most of the year, except for during the summer months, the UV index does not get high enough. Furthermore, getting sunlight from behind glass while indoors is not good for raising vitamin D levels, as glass filters out UVB rays, the ones responsible for making vitamin D.[12]

Overexposure to sunlight may increase the odds of developing certain skin cancers, especially in those whose skin tends to burn rather than tan in the sun.[13] You can protect yourself with sunscreen if you plan on spending more time in the sun; however, sunscreens may not be as safe as we thought, and some have toxic ingredients.[14] Do your research and buy safe brands. Or do what I recommend: if you are starting to burn, get out of the sun; you have made enough vitamin D for the day. If you must stay in the sun because you work outdoors, use protective barriers such as hats and UV protective clothing.

The best food sources for vitamin D include salmon, herring, halibut, sardines, trout, and cod liver oils. Small amounts of vitamin D are found in cheese, egg yolks, fortified milk, and cereals.[15] Mushrooms grown in sunlight or irradiated with UV light have a small amount of vitamin D_2, the weaker cousin of D_3. If you plan on supplementing, have your blood levels tested and get the recommendation of a professional. Getting too much vitamin D through supplementation can create toxic levels in the body.

3: Shop Strategically

We are now aware of the direct connection between certain chemicals in our products and their carcinogenic properties. I have mentioned this several times because it is one of the primary reasons for the rise in cancer rates. What can you do? Be vigilant with what you consume, and fast regularly. If you do these two things, you can greatly reduce your chance of developing cancer in your lifetime. Furthermore, if you follow all the suggestions in this book, you are way ahead of the curve.

4: Sugar, Sugar Everywhere

It is nearly impossible to escape this addictive substance. But that is precisely what we need to do to prevent cancer. Set up your life to avoid this sweet enemy. The best way is to not invite him into your home. When shopping at the grocery store, avoid going in the center aisles; that is where all the goodies with sugar hide. If buying boxed products, look at the ingredients list. If sugar/

fructose/sucrose or one of its many other derivatives, such as dextrose or maltose, is one of the first three ingredients, put the product back. The same goes for artificial sweeteners, such as aspartame and sucralose. The longer you and your family go without sweetened foods, the more you will appreciate the natural sweetness of regular foods, and your cravings will also reduce.

5: Food as Medicine

Include the following cancer-preventing foods in your diet:

- Garlic: Crush the garlic and let it sit for at least fifteen minutes to release allicin, the active compound. Organic garlic is better, and consuming it fresh and raw will provide the most benefits. However, cooking it minimally is also beneficial. Furthermore, studies on aged garlic extract show promise in reducing cancer.[16,17]
- Green tea:[18] Get it organic if you can, or go with the Japanese varieties. Drink two to three cups daily to get its benefits. Brewing the perfect cup of green tea is an art unto itself, however; boil the water and add it to a teapot with the tea leaves in it. Let it sit for two to three minutes to allow infusion and serve. The longer the infusion time, the more bitter the tea gets.
- Beets or beetroots: Just like garlic, beets have amazing cancer-preventing properties. The best way to eat them is to steam them for ten to fifteen minutes to extract the most nutrition.[19]
- Turmeric: Research is starting to prove how valuable this yellow root from the ginger family is.[20] The anticancer effects of curcumin, the active ingredient in turmeric, result from multiple biochemical mechanisms.[21] To get the therapeutic dose of turmeric, add half a teaspoon with a pinch of pepper to boiled milk and mix properly; once it cools a bit, add a little honey to taste and have it as a night-time drink before bed.
- Cruciferous vegetables, such as arugula, bok choy, broccoli, cabbage, cauliflower, and collard greens are cancer preventative and more bioavailable when lightly steamed or cooked.[22,23]
- Resveratrol, a powerful antioxidant, can prevent cancer growth. It is found mainly in red grapes, blueberries, cocoa, and peanuts. Select organic versions of these foods to get the most benefits.[24,25]

6: Therapeutic Fasting, the Great Healer

I left the best for last. In the detox section, we discussed fasting as an aid to detoxification, but I want to help you appreciate how powerful this practice is in preventing cancer.

As far back as the 1920s, scientists have been exploring the benefits of reducing calories by skipping meals. During that time, they found that significantly reducing calories helped mice live longer, healthier lives. Other researchers have found that in mice and monkeys, decreasing calorie consumption by 30 percent extended their life span by a third or more.[26] And in humans, improvements in the biomarkers for longevity are starting to be seen.[27] Although fasting diets have been criticized by nutritionists and other authorities, research suggests that prolonged fasting, longer than forty-eight hours, kick-starts stem cells into producing more white blood cells, which fight off cancer cells.[28]

This discovery could be particularly beneficial for those suffering from damaged immune systems, such as cancer patients on chemotherapy. It could also help the elderly, whose immune systems have become less effective. Another case series report showed that for those who are doing chemotherapy to fight cancer, fasting makes the cancer cells more receptive to the chemo drugs while keeping the healthy cells unharmed, and fasting helped in reducing fatigue and gastrointestinal side effects.[29]

Every day, we fast unknowingly for eight to ten hours when we sleep; hence, the word *breakfast* is used for the first meal of the day. This type of fasting is called intermittent fasting, because one has reduced or eliminated food intake for a short period of time. The benefit to this type of fasting comes once the glycogen (sugar) reserves in our liver and muscles are used up at night. This forces your body to go into ketosis to burn fat for energy. Once the body runs out of its primary source of fuel (glucose), it turns to alternate sources of energy. It starts digesting and breaking down dead or infected tissue and abnormal cells such as cancer cells for energy, basically cleaning house of unwanted things. Extending your nightly fast for an additional six to eight hours and breaking your fast around lunchtime will give your body small amounts of time every day to run these maintenance processes. In essence, you will be eating two main meals with a snack in between, if needed, during a smaller time window of approximately seven to eight hours a day, and fasting for the remaining time. Most of my patients find that doing intermittent fasting three to five days a week is a more manageable type of fasting for day-to-day living.

Once you are comfortable with these mini fasts and your body has become efficient at ketosis, you can attempt a longer twenty-four- to thirty-six-hour fast over the weekend or the days when you won't be busy. You should drink plenty of pure water during this time to keep your hydration levels steady, more than what you would drink normally, since you are compensating for the water intake not taken from food. I would suggest drinking no- or low-calorie drinks, such as herbal teas, as well. During this regeneration time, your body temperature may fall to conserve energy. Drinking ginger or cinnamon tea will help to warm you up. On occasion, you may get extreme hunger pangs or a headache, especially in the beginning. Eating a handful of nuts will save your sanity and not throw you out of ketosis. Once you break your fast, don't eat animal meat right away. Give your digestive system a couple of vegetarian meals to get up to speed before you assault it with a mountain of work in digesting meat. I generally don't recommend people do fasts longer than three days on their own. Longer fasts should be done under the care of a knowledgeable health practitioner. Doing a thirty-six-hour fast once a month with intermittent fasting of sixteen hours for three to five days a week will do amazing things for your health. In addition to this or by itself, you may do a seventy-two-hour or a three-day fast every change of season, or four times a year. How much or how little you fast will depend on your circumstance and tolerance level.

Once you start to see the benefits of fasting, you will have more motivation to fast regularly. Don't forget that our ancestors would fast not by choice, but because of lack of food. Because of this lifestyle behavior spanning thousands of years, our biology is programmed to function optimally with short periods of feasts followed by longer periods of fasts. I have focused on the benefit of fasting for cancer prevention, but the renewing and regenerative effects of fasting will have positive outcomes throughout your physical and mental states.

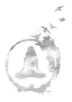

RULES FOR *Weight Management*

This chapter is not about a quick weight-loss strategy. Sorry to disappoint you, but it is true: you cannot have your cake and eat it too. Unless you are among the select few who can eat anything and not gain an ounce, maintaining a healthy weight into your golden years can become a challenge. However, there are solutions that work. Before we delve into weight management, we need to address what is considered a healthy weight. There are many formulas that calculate your ideal weight, of which one of the most recognized is the BMI (body mass index), which takes your height and weight into account, with any value over 30 considered obese. We want to avoid being in the obese category, since that is when most health problems start creeping up on you.[1] In general, BMI is a good indicator of healthy weight, as it gives you a range to fall into; however, its calculations lose efficacy for very muscular individuals, such as body builders, who would fall into the overweight or obese category because muscle weighs more than fat. So take all these formulas and calculators with a grain of salt.

The goal of this chapter is not about you becoming skinny, although you will get leaner by following the advice here. It is more about you reaching and maintaining a body composition of muscle and fat that will allow for a healthy metabolism, balanced hormones, and overall wellness. If you are following all the recommendations in this book and still gaining weight, then there could be an underlying medical issue, such as hypothyroidism or Cushing's syndrome. Your doctor can do the appropriate tests to figure out the cause and treat it. Medications such as beta-blockers[2] and antidepressants[3] can also make you gain weight. If you suspect your medication is making you gain weight, ask your doctor for an effective alternative that won't add on the pounds. Never stop or change any medication regimen without consulting your physician.

Most of us gain weight because of our diet and lifestyle. Let me elucidate: humans have evolved for most of our existence to be hunters and gatherers, and having such a lifestyle meant we didn't have regular access to food as we do now. Instead, when we had food available, we would eat a lot and store it as fat to be used for energy on the days and weeks we didn't have food. Fast-forward now, and the situation has changed, but the genes responsible for energy storage and metabolism haven't caught up yet. With the advent of modern manufacturing processes and supermarkets on almost every corner, we have access to lots of calorie-dense foods all the time. We gorge ourselves every day with large portions of food; combine that with our sedentary lifestyle, and we have a recipe for easy storage of fat. We panic at the thought of skipping a meal, fearing it will damage our metabolism. But rest assured it won't.[4] We cannot change our DNA overnight, but we can adjust how we eat to more closely resemble how our ancestors ate.

Why am I emphasizing our diet rather than exercise when it comes to weight management? Most of your weight is determined by the food you eat, as well as how and when you eat it. Although exercise is important in many aspects of health, it is not a very effective tool for weight loss if you don't manage your diet well. Exercise will raise your metabolism for a few hours, but it will also make you hungrier, and some folks can justify eating unhealthy, calorie-dense foods after a workout only to be disappointed later on. We cannot have an effective long-term food plan if we count every calorie; it is tedious and ineffective. For something to be effective, it needs to be relatively quick, easy, and efficient.

The following are a few suggestions that will work if you stick with them:

1: Take Back Your Kitchen

One of the biggest culprits in our battle of the bulge is the simple carbohydrates found in processed foods and derivatives of refined grains. We have become such a fast-everything society, no one has the patience to do anything slowly and right. Fast food is designed to be cheap and tasty. It is dense with simple carbs and unhealthy fats and loaded with elements to make it taste good. Real, wholesome food is more expensive and takes time to prepare. It is more nutritious, has a plethora of healthy ingredients, and has a more balanced portfolio of carbs, proteins, and fats. What do I mean when I say *real food*? It is food that comes straight from the farm into your kitchen, most times via the farmers' market. It has zero processing done to it in factories.

Simple carbs such as chips, cookies, sweets, cakes, and other pastries, although delicious, are undeniably our Achilles' heel. Nearly no one is immune to them. It is not that they are inherently bad, but they can easily become adverse because we have continuous access to them. They are meant to be consumed in small amounts, on occasion, and as a treat, not after every meal as a dessert or when you sit to watch TV or when you are bored or when there is no food to eat. You get what I am saying. If this just described your eating habits, then here is the solution that will change your life.

- First, look in your kitchen cupboards, pantry, or wherever you hide your goodies, and collect them all. Every single one of them. You know by now which products I am talking about. It is the stuff that makes you feel ashamed after eating it. The highly processed foods with high sugar, fat, or salt content. You can either donate them to the food bank or give them to friends and family. I don't like throwing away edible food, but if you want, you can throw these foods away.

- The next time you go food shopping, eat a meal before you go. When you shop on a full stomach, you won't be tempted to pick up junk food. To your best ability, buy all the wholesome foods we talked about in the food chapter. Now that your house has only healthy food, try your best to keep it that way. It will be a challenge if you have kids and a partner in the house who are providing resistance. They may unwittingly sabotage your weight loss efforts by bringing home junk food. You need to be patient and allow some time for this transition by educating them on why you are making this change.

- Designate one day a week where you allow yourself to eat anything you want, within moderation, of course. This will be your cheat day. However, I don't like how it implies that you are doing something bad, which you are not, so we will call it something more positive, like "Happy Belly Day," or whatever name you want to give it. This way you won't feel like you are depriving yourself. On this chosen day, get the appropriate amount of junk food, enough for one day, and consume it. You are not going to store it for another day. If you are going to a party and you know there will be cakes and cookies and other goodies there, then designate that day your Happy Belly Day.

2: Eat When You Are Hungry

The concept of eating three square meals a day is not based on science or our metabolic needs but is a cultural construct left over from when early European settlers thought it was more civilized to have timed meals, compared to the natives who ate in varied patterns depending on the seasons.[5] You don't need to eat three meals a day or even five small meals to keep a healthy weight. The best way to gauge whether you are ready to eat is to listen to your body's cues. Eat when you feel hungry, not when you think you must eat. If the thought of food doesn't make your mouth salivate, you are not hungry yet. Remember the last time you were truly hungry? What signals did your body give you? Was it an empty feeling in your throat and stomach, or was it a loud growl? Did you feel lightheaded or become easily agitated? Whatever signals you got, that is what you need to rely on to eat, because that is when your body is truly ready to accept food. For some individuals, it may take five hours to get these signals, while some may go twelve hours until they feel hungry. Once you start eating when you are truly hungry, you may notice that you don't retain as much fat as you used to and you can digest your food better.

3: Tackle Your Food Intolerances

You will know something you are consuming is not good for you by how you feel after consuming it. You may feel lethargic and have a harder time focusing, or your digestion may get impaired and you may have chronic bloating. Your hormones may get imbalanced, and you could have a harder time losing weight. Most times you may crave the very foods you are intolerant to. Whatever you feel will be unique to you. Paying attention to how you feel after eating or drinking something is a good habit to form. It will give you useful information you can use later to make decisions about your food choices. Sometimes, the unpleasant symptoms will have a time delay and may happen in the next day or two, which will make it more difficult to pinpoint which foods are the culprits.

If you have multiple food sensitivities, then doing something like an elimination diet followed by a challenge protocol under the supervision of a professional will be helpful in identifying your intolerances. I will describe how the process works. We have alluded to this previously, but to properly do this protocol, you need to eliminate any foods you suspect may be an issue from your diet completely for at least one month. The most common foods eliminated are gluten-containing foods, such as wheat, rye, barley, and bulgur. Also, dairy, soy, eggs, shellfish, corn, peanuts and tree nuts, caffeine, alcohol, refined sugar (and products containing it), chocolate, artificial colors and flavors, and sometimes nightshade vegetables, such as tomatoes, potatoes, bell peppers, and eggplants. Depending on how serious your case is, you may need to eliminate all of these or a portion. During the month you are off these foods, you need to be careful not to have any of them unknowingly by reading product labels carefully and minimize eating out. Otherwise, you may get mixed results. The best way is to make food at home, where you will have control over what you prepare and eat. I know this is hard and a lot of my patients have complained about it, but it is the gold standard in identifying food intolerances. Think of the health benefits you will get and the years of relief from all the unpleasant symptoms and possible health issues you can avoid by doing it right. That is why I recommended that you see a professional to get the support you might need. Since for most of us the foods on the elimination list form a big part of our diet, you will be forced to expand your palate and discover new foods to eat, which is a good thing. Keep a journal and notice any changes in yourself during this time. Have your aches and pains reduced or disappeared? Has your eczema cleared up? Are you getting good bowel movements now? How is your mood or energy?

Once you are ready to reintroduce the eliminated foods into your diet, start by eating the food you suspect you are least sensitive to for at least one day or three meals, and see if your symptoms return. I would keep foods containing gluten and dairy for the end, since a lot of people react to them. Keeping a food journal will help during this discovery phase. If a reintroduced food does not cause any issues, it may be left in the diet. You can move on to another food. If a food you ate gave you unpleasant symptoms, then you may need to remove it from your diet permanently. Give your digestive system a couple of days to reduce its inflammation. During this time, go back to your elimination diet until your gut has healed, and then reintroduce the next food and so on until you have reintroduced all the foods. Well done! You have identified your food intolerances! Try your best not to eat the foods you are intolerant to for at least six months to a year, and watch how your body heals itself. At a later date, you may try the challenge protocol again to see if you can eat the foods you are sensitive to without eliciting symptoms. In rare cases, this is possible, but most likely you will get a reaction, and a choice has to be made whether you want to keep the food in your diet and suffer the consequences or remove it for the remainder of your life and be healthier. This is a hard decision, but it's doable if you can reengineer your lifestyle to reduce the odds of running into that food. The easiest way is to not bring the offending foods into your home, so you are not tempted to eat them, and to do research beforehand when eating out. More and more restaurants offer gluten- and dairy-free options. You can also ask them not to include certain ingredients in your meal. With time, this will become second nature, and you won't miss the foods that were hurting you.

4: Intermittent Fasting 101

We have discussed fasting in great length, and we touched upon intermittent fasting; however, that was in the context of helping the body remove toxins efficiently and to renew and regenerate your body. Another great benefit of intermittent fasting is its positive effect on metabolism, inflammation, and weight loss.[6,7] Doing the 16-8 protocol, where you would fast for a period of sixteen hours and eat within an eight-hour window during a twenty-four-hour period, has become popular for good reason, because it works. In this scenario, the simplest way to do it would be to skip your first meal of the day and eat the remaining two meals within an eight-hour window. For example, if you sleep by 10 p.m. and wake up by 7 a.m., then your first meal would be at noon, and your last meal would be before 8 p.m. Start by doing this protocol three days a week for the first month, and then add on days until you reach an equilibrium, where you are happy with the results. As with any new dietary changes, your body will need a little time adjusting. Staying hydrated is the key in this transition.

To prevent energy-level fluctuation that can happen initially because of low blood sugar, drink small amounts of apple cider vinegar as needed, about a teaspoon to a tablespoon each time, with some water. This will help keep your blood sugar steady and energy levels constant.[8,9,10] If you like cinnamon, another great blood sugar regulator,[11] you can sprinkle a small amount of cinnamon powder on your meals to a max of half a teaspoon a day. Alternatively, you can drink cinnamon tea. Boil a couple of cinnamon sticks in water for ten to fifteen minutes. Turn off the stove and wait a short while for the color to release, and then slowly sip and enjoy.

Losing weight properly takes time. Take it day by day, and consider eating a Mediterranean-type diet to supplement your weight-loss goals.

5: Eat a Mediterranean-Type Diet

This food-choice regimen places an emphasis on fresh fruits and vegetables, with healthy plant-based fats and fish for protein. Out of all the diets out there, this is one of the best and most sustainable. Here are the basics:

- **Eat mostly:** non-starchy fruits and vegetables, seafood, healthy fats, legumes, nuts, seeds, whole grains, and herbs and spices
- **Eat moderately:** eggs, cheese, and yogurt
- **Eat occasionally:** poultry and red meat[12]

6: Ketogenic Diet to the Rescue

If losing fat and maintaining a healthy weight is a challenge, you may be able to overcome this obstacle by following the ketogenic diet for a period of three to six months. It is a high-fat, moderate protein, and low-carb diet. This diet was invented as an aid for patients with epilepsy, as it reduced their symptoms.[13] However, it seems to help reduce the risk of neurodegenerative diseases as well.[14] One of the beneficial side effects of this diet is weight loss.[15] Essentially, a ketogenic diet puts your body into ketosis, a metabolic state where most of the body's energy comes from ketones, a product of fat breakdown. When you're following a ketogenic diet, your body is burning fat for energy rather than carbohydrates. Our bodies mainly run on glucose for energy. Ordinarily, we have eight to twelve hours of it stored in our liver and muscles as glycogen. Once it's no longer available, we begin to burn our stored fat. Like fasting, which puts you into ketosis, a ketogenic diet limits the carbohydrates you consume, with most of your calories coming from fats. By eating this way, you train your body to burn fat for energy.

There are various forms of ketogenic diets. I recommend you stick with the standard ketogenic diet, which puts a high emphasis on healthy fats as the main source of fuel. If you find this too challenging, you may bump up your protein intake by lowering your fat intake. You can do a search on meal plans for ketogenic diets to get a better idea of how to incorporate it into your day. Some folks like the ketogenic diet because it allows them to eat bacon and pork and other high-fat meats they enjoy. I would caution on getting your fat intake from such sources, as they can raise your bad cholesterol. Instead, opt for plant- or fish-based fats as much as possible.

The following are foods you can include on a ketogenic diet:

- **Avocados:** or avocado dishes like guacamole
- **Fatty fish:** trout, anchovies, sardines, salmon, and mackerel
- **Healthy oils:** mainly coconut oil, avocado oil, and virgin olive oil
- **Cheese:** unprocessed cheese (goat, cottage, blue, or cheddar)
- **Butter and cream:** grass fed when possible or made from goat/sheep milk
- **Meat:** steak, chicken, and turkey
- **Eggs:** free-range, cage-free, or organic eggs
- **Yogurt:** Greek yogurt and full-fat yogurt
- **Nuts and seeds:** Walnuts, almonds, pistachios, flax seeds, pumpkin seeds, chia seeds, and hemp seeds
- **Low-carb veggies:** most green veggies, cucumbers, mushrooms, green beans, asparagus, cauliflower, kale, broccoli, celery, tomatoes, onions, peppers, and brussels sprouts
- **Low-carb fruits in moderation:** apricots, peaches, plums, cherries, cantaloupe, grapefruit, strawberries, blackberries, raspberries, olives, coconuts, and lemons
- **Herbs and spices** (most spices are low in carbs; use the following for added weight-loss benefit): cayenne pepper, turmeric, cinnamon, garlic, ginger, black pepper, basil, dill, oregano, rosemary, thyme, and nutmeg

Initially, going on a ketogenic diet may create uncomfortable symptoms. Low energy, brain fog, and digestive issues are quite common and may last a few days. If the symptoms are intolerable, increase your carb intake slightly for a couple of weeks until your symptoms subside, and then go back to your original diet. There will be shifts in your body's electrolytes and mineral balance as well.[16] Use a good-quality sea salt and take a magnesium supplement to offset this imbalance. Increasing your coconut oil intake may also help alleviate the unpleasant symptoms. Please let your doctor know that you have gone on this type of diet so that he or she can monitor your health more closely, especially if you plan to do this long term. This is just as a precaution; every individual's biochemistry is different.

My goal is to help you appreciate what these food choices can do to help you with your weight-loss and weight-management goals, with foundational knowledge of what these diets entail. Depending on what you decide to do, inform yourself adequately before delving in to help minimize unfavorable outcomes that could arise and to maximize the effects of the diet. I am quite certain that whether you choose to go on the Mediterranean diet or the ketogenic diet or any combination of food choices along with intermittent fasting and all the other suggestions thus far, you will improve your body composition and create a leaner, healthier frame.

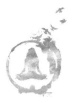

TWELVE WEEKS TO *Optimum Health*

I hope you have found the material in this book helpful thus far. Since a lot of information and lifestyle suggestions have been presented, it may be a predicament to decide what to do and how to go about doing it. The choice is up to you. Look at how healthy you are and your current lifestyle, and based on what we have discussed, decide which areas could use improvement. The more changes you can make, the better, but even a few small adjustments should result in an improvement in your health. Use this section to help start your journey into optimum health.

To provide structure and to gradually bring about change in your lifestyle and dietary behaviors, I have broken down what you need to do on a week-by-week basis to effectively reach optimum health. I use this method with my patients, and they find it much easier to implement with higher compliance and success rates. Every week, you will continue what you had started the previous weeks, while implementing the current week's protocols. Some folks may need more time to adjust, and that is okay. If you find a particular week more challenging, give yourself additional time before continuing. If you are already doing a particular week's recommendation, move on to the next week, and you will finish even sooner. I would recommend keeping a journal or weekly planner and logging the changes you are making on a daily and weekly basis to keep you accountable and more motivated. You may also note any physical, mental, and emotional improvements. This will help you connect which dietary and lifestyle behaviors were the underlying cause for the ailments you were experiencing.

Before proceeding, make sure you have read all the chapters until this point, as you will have to refer to them. It will be easier to go back to them and know where to focus if you have already read them.

Week 1: We will begin this week with breathing right. Start by doing the belly breathing you learned in the chapter on air. Do this while you are sleeping to help you learn it more effectively, always making sure that your exhalation is longer than your inhalation. Spend five minutes twice daily focusing on breathing right. This would constitute about twenty-five to thirty breaths each time. You can start with ten breaths and build up from there, if you like.

I recommend doing it before sleeping and on waking to make things easier. If you are a smoker, this is the time you commit to quitting for life.

Week 2: This is going to be hydration week. You are going to fall in love with water this week. Following the rules in the water chapter, drink enough water to make your urine colorless most of the time. Some folks like to sip on water throughout the day, and others like to chug a couple of glasses every few hours. Do what works for you. If the taste of water is unappealing, then add a slice of organic lemon to your water to improve the taste. To save time, you can preslice the lemons and freeze them in a container, using them as needed.

Week 3: For the next three weeks, we will be focusing on what you eat. This week you are going to increase your vegetable and fruit intake. Go grocery shopping and get a variety of fruits and veggies of all different colors. Eat two to three pieces of fruit daily. If incorporating the vegetables into your dishes, then half your plate should be veggies. On the days that you eat meat or fewer vegetables, have a large salad for one of your meals. A favorite salad of mine is one with tomatoes, cucumber, radishes, red onions, yellow or orange bell peppers, zucchini, and cilantro. You can make a meal out of the salad by adding cooked beans, such as black or pinto beans, or a couple of boiled eggs with a sprinkle of feta or cottage cheese. For dressing, make your own simple dressing with two parts olive oil to one part balsamic vinegar and honey to taste. I like to add yellow mustard paste as well for the added flavor. Play around with the ingredients until you find a combination that works for you.

Week 4: For this week, we will aim to reduce your sweetened food consumption. If you like to have dessert after your meals or eat snacks of chocolate, cookies, and other pastries, then let's replace them with a healthier alternative. For example, consider satisfying your sweet tooth with dates, raisins, or other dried fruits, such as prunes, figs, and apricots. If you still need to have chocolate, go for the darker varieties. Eat everything in moderation. Don't sit with the whole bag. Put a few pieces on a small plate and take that with you to eat; you will eat less this way. While you are changing over to healthier alternatives, consider removing all the unhealthy sweets and pastries from your house.

Week 5: This week we will build up your gut microbiome by increasing your probiotic consumption. Pick at least three forms of fermented foods from products such as yogurt, kefir, miso, natto, tempeh, sauerkraut, kimchi, pickles, and kombucha, and eat these with your meals as a side dish or drink, gradually increasing their consumption. Be ready for extra gas production this week. For additional guidance, refer to "Probiotics 101" in the food chapter.

Week 6: We will focus on stress management this week. As you have worked on improving your breathing these past few weeks, you may have noticed an improvement in your stress response. Let's take it a step further and start meditating for five minutes every day this week. Please refer to the meditation section of the stress-management chapter. If you are having a hard time focusing on your breath while seated, my suggestion is to start with walking meditation. Pay attention to how your feet touch the ground while you walk and the sensations produced in your legs. Later, you can move on to paying attention to sounds, smells, or sights around you, focusing on one sensation at a time. Find a quiet place, and walk back and forth slowly while doing this type of meditation. The following weeks, you can try going back to seated meditation and gradually increase your meditation time by five minutes each week until you can do half an hour daily. There is no hard-and-fast rule with meditation. Find what works for you. You may even break it up into two or more shorter sessions during the day to suit your lifestyle and stress-management needs.

Week 7: We will incorporate more movement this week. You can do this by walking at a moderate pace for half an hour daily or, at the least, every other day. Try to walk fast enough that your breathing gets quicker, but not so fast that you cannot hold a conversation with someone because of breathlessness. Also take this opportunity to get as much sunlight as you can. Don't burn your skin from excess sun exposure, though. You may also join a gym and do more conventional exercises, but, at the minimum, walk on a treadmill or elliptical machine for half an hour. If gravity is an issue and your knees or hips hurt, then consider swimming. I want you to be thinking about how you can move more throughout this week. You could get an app on your phone to remind you to move whenever you are sedentary.

Week 8: Let's work on sleep this week. What I find most with my patients is how little they sleep and still manage to function, albeit suboptimally. Let's aim to get at minimum 7.5 hours of sleep daily, ideally nine hours. If you have been getting just five or six hours of sleep, then increase it by half-hour increments each week until you reach my recommendation. Follow the suggestions in the sleep chapter to improve the quality of your sleep as well.

Week 9: This week, we will embrace our emotions. You will work on your relationships with loved ones and friends and heal any that need healing. Take your time. Go through the chapter on relationships and prioritize the relationships that need your most and immediate attention.

Week 10: This is going to be brain-challenge week. You are going to sharpen your mind by adopting brain-improvement habits. Read the chapter on healthy mind and incorporate some of the suggestions into your life, even if it's just one thing, such as doing a word puzzle. Try a few of the suggestions to figure out what you like and spend time every day training your mind to stay fit into your golden years.

Week 11: Now that you have prepared your body and mind, it's time to go to the next phase, which is to detoxify. Following the recommendations in the detoxification chapter, try your best to remove or reduce the toxins from your immediate environment, and start doing the detoxification recommendations on a daily and weekly basis.

Week 12: Last, we will invoke one of the great healers: fasting. We will start with intermittent fasting as described in the cancer-prevention and weight-management chapter. Do the 16-8 protocol for three days this week, and see how you feel. Continue the intermittent fasting if you feel it's something you can manage on a long-term basis. If not, consider doing a twenty-four-hour fast once a month to help you detoxify and heal.

At the end of twelve weeks, or whenever you finish, assess yourself. Have you reached a point where you are happy with your health outcome and the results you are getting? Are there things you need to work more on? You might spend additional time mastering those elements. Look back on the things you have accomplished in the past twelve weeks. Congratulate yourself on your dedication and know that you have positively influenced your health. Continue by making these healthy lifestyle behaviors a part of your life, and watch the magic happen.

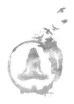

RULES FOR *Healthy Pregnancy*

Having someone grow inside you is a big deal. As mothers-to-be, there are certain expectations society puts on you, like how you should conduct yourself in every aspect of your pregnancy, from baby showers to baby clothes. There can be tremendous pressures put on you, which can be unfair at times. We need to deal with everyday uncertainties, but instead of diluting your mind with unnecessary stress, try your best to focus on providing a nurturing environment for your growing baby.

As always, my emphasis is on a holistic approach, and with pregnancy, it is no different. This chapter will focus on maintaining a healthy pregnancy from preconception to postpartum.

1: Planning Starts Way before Getting Pregnant

As with any major decision in life, bringing a child into this world requires careful planning and preparation. This is no time to be spontaneous, at least not in this day and age. First and foremost, you need to ask yourself why you want a baby. The answer may surprise you. Your life partner should also answer this question. Is it to solidify the union of your marriage by bringing a symbol of your love for each other into this world, or is it because all your friends already had a baby? Maybe your parents are pressuring you for a grandchild or there is emptiness in the relationship that you hope a baby will fill. Whatever the answer, it needs to feel right for you. Are you and your partner on the same wavelength? Is your relationship healthy and stable? If not, you might work on that before considering pregnancy.

Once you are certain you want a child, you should determine if your life is set up to welcome a child. Are your financials in order? Babies are expensive. Do you have money saved for emergencies? If not, you better start saving, even if it's just a few dollars every week. Make sure your living situation and your career are where you want them to be for the next few years. This is no time to make big changes and put yourself under unnecessary stress once you are pregnant. All this preparation should happen months before trying to get pregnant.

Other things to do and consider:

- Making sure you are physically healthy before getting pregnant is crucial. If you are overweight or obese, try to lose at least 10 percent of your body mass to improve your odds of conceiving and having a healthier pregnancy.[1] If you are infertile, include exercise along with a healthy diet as part of your health strategy, as it has shown to improve fertility.[2] But keep in mind that intense physical activity in women may interfere with the menstrual cycle and decrease fertility.[3]
- Give yourself at least three to six months to detox your body before trying to conceive, and remove as many toxic products as you can from your immediate surroundings by following the advice in this book.
- Start eating more fruits, green leafy vegetables, and safe, oily fish to load up on the nutrient reserves in your body. As an assurance, take a good-quality prenatal vitamin and mineral supplement with B vitamins, especially folate (vitamin B_9) and B_{12}.
- Get as much direct sunlight as you can (within safety limits, of course) to boost your vitamin D stores. Also get in as much sleep as you can to help you through this transition in your life. You may not be able to get regular quality sleep once the baby comes.
- If you are taking medication for a health condition, consult your physician to make sure their use will be safe during pregnancy, and if not, switch to a safer option.
- Get a vaginal swab to rule out low-grade infections that may lead to preterm delivery. It may also be a good time to consider screening for inherited genetic disorders for both you and your partner. If there is a possibility of passing on a devastating disease to your unborn child, some hard decisions need to be made. I think it's better to make these decisions before trying to conceive, as you can have more informed choices, such as using a sperm donor or even adoption.
- Although we can never predict life events, you want to do your best to be in a tranquil state when trying to conceive. Stress may affect a woman's chances of getting pregnant,[4] and in men it has shown to decrease semen quality.[5] If you are a particularly stressed individual trying to conceive, then make it a habit to practice meditation regularly, along with the other relaxation skills you have discovered in this book.

2: Pregnancy Dos and Don'ts

Pregnancy is a wonderful and scary adventure. Your body will be ready to do its thing, but your mind may be all over the place. It's okay and normal to be worried about everything. Educating yourself and your partner will minimize some of your anxiety and is the key to having a healthy pregnancy. There are many prenatal education programs and classes, some of them online. Choose the one that resonates with you. These education sessions will go through many areas related to pregnancy, such as changes your body will go through, things to avoid, and labor and birth preparation, as well as many of your concerns as a parent-to-be. Make a list of all your questions and go prepared. Although you will be quite well prepared through these prenatal classes, there are some strategic details I want to emphasize.

- Remember that because you are a vessel for your growing child, your baby will sample whatever you put in your body. This is not a time to eat whatever you want. Eat clean and modestly and increase calorie consumption slightly when moving toward the second and third trimester. Make sure you are following the rules in this book, paying special attention to the first six chapters. Listen to your body and give it what it needs. During this time, women become more intuitive to their needs. Find comfort in this intelligent design. When you crave something, satisfy it, but also be mindful not to overindulge.

- Smoking and drinking alcohol are an absolute no-no. Smoking is linked to low birth weights.[6] Also, stay away from people while they smoke. Alcohol is linked to fetal alcohol syndrome, a group of symptoms leading to physical and behavioral limitations in the child.[7] Not even a small amount is considered safe. If you love your coffee or tea, cut back considerably,[8] or even better, try to avoid it while pregnant. Your baby will thank you.

- Don't change cat litter or handle garden soil during your pregnancy. If you must, wear gloves. Toxoplasmosis, although rare, can affect the baby and lead to blindness and other neurological concerns.[9]

- Don't eat raw or undercooked vegetables or meats, including fish, or deli meat and soft cheeses made from unpasteurized milk.[10] This advice is meant as a precaution and not to frighten you. You don't need to obsess about what you eat, but being aware will lower the odds of anything serious happening.

- Try to eat lightly cooked and warm food for most of your meals to reduce the burden on your digestive system. Eating more soups and stews during this time will help your body assimilate more nutrients. According to traditional Chinese medicine, eating warm foods will boost the body's blood and qi and direct these energies to the lower abdomen and reproductive organs.[11]

- Get routine checkups with your doctor and have a health-care team you can rely on. If you want to go for a more holistic route, you will want a midwife or doula on your team. Get your blood and urine work done early and ask for a complete thyroid panel, iron stores, and B$_{12}$ levels. Thyroid hormone is critical for brain development in the baby, and mothers with thyroid deficiency have shown to have children with lower IQ scores.[12] Make sure your thyroid hormones are within normal levels, and if they are not, get it treated right away. Furthermore, conditions like gestational diabetes and preeclampsia are manageable if caught early on.

- Prepare your body and your uterus for delivering your bundle of joy. One way is to work on the pelvic floor muscles with exercises that target them; their proper functioning will help as the pregnancy progresses. The well-known Kegel exercise strengthens the pelvic floor muscles. However, I believe the reverse Kegel, used to stretch and relax the pelvic floor muscles, may be just as important. These practices have been shown to reduce incontinence and lead to a shorter and smoother labor.[13,14] I recommend that you educate yourself before doing these exercises and even consider consulting a professional such as a physiotherapist who specializes in pelvic floor muscles if you think this is an area you need to work on.

- Another trick used by midwives is to suggest drinking red raspberry–leaf tea during the last trimester. This ritual aims to tone the uterus and help it work more efficiently during labor. Since there isn't much research behind its efficacy and safety,[15] I would use it optimistically but with caution. If you do decide to use it, a sensible approach would be to start slowly toward the end of pregnancy, around the thirty-two- to thirty-four-week mark, by drinking a cup or two of the tea daily. If you notice strong Braxton Hicks contractions, then cut back how much you are drinking.

- Write a birth plan. You have read books about pregnancy and taken prenatal classes and spoken to other moms. You have developed a good grasp of the entire process and what to expect. Now is the time to reflect on how you want the birth process to play out and write it down. Anything from what music you want to be playing to what position you want to deliver in; you should note the kind of pain relief you want, if any, and if you want to breastfeed or bottle-feed. Nothing is off the table. This is your birth plan. Focus on what is important to you, and don't just go with what others have done. Communicate this plan to your health-care team so they know your wishes, but be aware that circumstances may change and your midwife or doctor may have to do what's best for you and the baby even if it's not something you had asked for. Having a doula or a supportive partner next to you who understands your birth plan lets them know what things are important to you, and they will try their best to make sure your wishes are carried out by being your advocate during a time when you may not be able to think clearly.

- Make being mindful a big part of your journey into motherhood. Your body and your emotions will go through changes during this transition. Use the belly-breathing technique you learned in this book to center yourself, especially when your mind is distracted and overwhelmed by emotions. Bring attention into your body and the sensations you feel. Being more aware will help guide you to make better decisions. Use the progressive relaxation technique we learned in the sleep chapter to relax your muscles, and scan your body regularly to identify trouble areas. Being mindful throughout your pregnancy will help you remember those precious moments and the wonderful feelings that come with them, things that cannot be captured on camera. Everyone will have an opinion about your pregnancy, but listen to your intuition as well, and trust in it to guide you. Have faith, and use the power of prayer, if you are so inclined, to get you through any difficult times.

3: Postpartum Advice

The first few weeks after giving birth is a time for you to heal and rejuvenate and get close to your baby. Depending on your physiology and how much energy went into your labor, whether you had a natural birth or a C-section, the time it takes for recovery will vary. You may have a lot of people wanting to congratulate you and meet the baby. It's okay to say no nicely and ask them to visit after a couple of weeks. Hopefully, you will have close family and friends who can lend a helping hand with household chores during this time. The last thing you want to worry about is doing the laundry or cooking food. Ask for help. It doesn't make you weak. It makes you smart. All you should worry about for the first few weeks is feeding your baby and taking care of yourself.

Your pelvic floor muscles and all the adjoining areas will be sore initially. Try a sitz bath to provide relief.[16] In this bath, you submerge your bottom in a shallow pool of warm water for about fifteen minutes. You can do it in a clean bathtub or buy a portable kit that fits over the toilet. You may add up to a half cup of Epsom salt to the bath for added relief. Cut back the salt if it stings. If there is considerable discomfort, then a cold sitz bath may be more beneficial for the first few days.[17] Do not sit in an ice-cold bath. Instead, add ice cubes to the water while seated to cool it gradually.[18]

Some other things may happen as well. Your uterus will still contract to return to normal, and you will bleed from time to time for the first few weeks. Peeing and pooping may be a challenge for a while. Urinary and sometimes bowel incontinence can be common for the first few weeks, and temporary loss of urine control when you cough or strain may occur.[19] Continue practicing your Kegel exercises to improve urinary incontinence. You may also experience constipation right after delivery.[20] Hydrate properly and have plenty of fiber in your diet to make your bowels soft and regular. Your sleep will be all over the place initially. Sleep whenever you get a chance. The best time is when your baby is asleep. You may be sad and cry more than usual for the first few days, and that is normal. Try to be patient with yourself, as you can get overwhelmed with all the responsibilities of a new baby. But if you are extremely sad or are unable to take care of your baby or yourself, you may have postpartum depression, and you should go see your doctor.[21] You may sweat more and smell different or more than usual, and that is normal too.[22] Skin and hair changes are also normal. If you had developed thicker hair during pregnancy, it may start to shed, and you may get more skin breakouts, dry patches, or pigmentation in the months following delivery.[23] Your body is going through hormonal fluctuations until a new norm is reached, and this is causing the changes you see.[24,25] Sleep and good nutrition are vital in helping you heal and for your hormones to balance. Relax and bond with your baby, and let your loved ones take care of you.

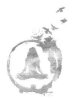

RULES FOR *Raising Healthy Kids*

L et me ask you this: What is the biggest impact we can have on future generations? I believe it is in how we raise the current generation. Our children will grow up to be our engineers, doctors, and policemen and women, all of whom provide valuable services to society. They will become lawyers and politicians and carve out the fate of their brethren. They will become parents themselves one day and raise future generations.

Parents want the best for their children. We want to raise healthy, happy, smart, and resilient children. Our goal as parents should be to raise kids who will not only grow up to become successful adults, but also altruistic visionaries who will make the world a better place. Raising healthy children means raising children who are not only healthy physically, but also emotionally and mentally. If you are a parent, this is one of the most important things you will do in your lifetime.

Every child is unique, and what works for one child may not work for another. The best judge of what will work for your child is your child's feedback to you through body language, verbal responses, and sometimes overt expressions. We can use empirical evidence and knowledge passed down through generations; however, it's usually a process of trial and error until you find what works. I will try my best to distill the most essential wisdom for you here.

1: The Miracle Baby Food

Let's start with one of the most important things you can do for your baby's health after he or she is born. Yes, I am talking about breastfeeding. Health experts believe that breast milk is the best natural food choice for babies, as it provides all the nutrients and energy a baby needs for the first few months of life.[1] Infant formula is considered as a healthy alternative.[2] How long a mother breastfeeds will depend on her circumstances and the child's needs. The World Health Organization recommends breastfeeding exclusively for the first six months and to continue breastfeeding while introducing other foods for up to two years or longer, as long as mother and child are willing.[3]

Breastfed babies have fewer infections and hospitalizations than formula-fed infants. Breast milk contains natural antibodies not found in commercial formulas, which helps strengthen your baby's immune system. This helps lower a baby's chances of getting many infections, including ear infections, respiratory infections, and allergies. Breastmilk is usually more easily digested than formula, which can create fewer bouts of constipation, diarrhea, or gas in the baby.[4] The American Academy of Pediatrics (AAP) points out that mothers who breastfeed their babies return to their prepregnancy weight sooner and have a decreased risk for breast and ovarian cancers.[5]

Sometimes, if the baby is not latching properly, he or she may not get enough milk, or the mother may not be producing enough milk. This may compel the mother to bottle-feed with formula, and that is okay. Feeding your child is more important than making sure he or she only gets breast milk. Although I have emphasized the importance of breast milk for the baby, the choice to feed formula or breast milk to your baby is up to you. It will depend on factors such as lifestyle, comfort, and whether you can breastfeed. Don't let anyone shame you into feeling guilty about your choice.

Once the child gets teeth and starts biting on the nipple, it may become uncomfortable to breastfeed, but don't get discouraged. There are techniques to overcome these situations. For example, breast milk can be pumped and frozen for later bottle-feeding, so just make sure to freeze and thaw properly. A lactation consultant is invaluable in such circumstances, and your doctor can help you get in contact with one. Also, if you find that you are producing more milk than your baby can consume, consider donating it to a human milk bank, which can help save preterm or sick babies in hospitals.

2: Peanut Allergies Debunked

When it comes to peanut allergies, new research has indicated that introducing peanut butter to your child before the first year may help reduce peanut allergies later. Peanut allergy can present itself as itching or tingling around the mouth and throat; skin reactions such as redness, swelling, and hives; or digestive problems such as stomach cramps, diarrhea, nausea, or vomiting. There could also be more serious anaphylaxis, such as swelling of the tongue and airway, trouble breathing, dizziness or fainting, and a rapid heart rate.[6] In the study, researchers looked at peanut allergies in infants. If the children had an allergic reaction to their first meal of peanuts, they were excluded from the study. However, for the majority of kids, early introduction to peanuts during the first year of life appeared to be beneficial at reducing the risk of developing an allergy to peanuts later on.[7] Furthermore, another study saw a tenfold reduction in peanut allergy in a population where infants consumed large quantities of peanuts in the first year of life, compared to a population that avoided it.[8] This is good news for parents who are afraid of giving peanuts to their children. Just a note of caution, though: if your child has never eaten peanuts before, be ready for the possibility of a serious anaphylactic reaction, which will require administration of epinephrine (adrenaline) through an auto-injector and a visit to the emergency room.[9] These reactions could happen to any foods and not just peanuts. I would introduce peanuts slowly, with a small amount at first, and watch for reactions. If there is any allergic reaction, then don't give your child peanuts at all. Otherwise, gradually increase their consumption of them and make them part of their diet.

3: Give Your Child a Break

Now that your child is growing and you are taking care of his or her physical needs, your focus might shift to their developmental needs and schooling. You may feel pressure to make sure your child reaches his or her full potential. So what do most parents do? They fill every available time slot with extra scholastic classes for their child to attend. The schools are not helping either by sending kids home with a large homework load, which only raises kids' stress levels, as well as yours if you think you cannot help them.[10] Plus, there is an increased risk for obesity in overly stressed children, especially for boys.[11] If this is the situation for your child, then try to figure out ways to alleviate his or her stress. You could get involved with the school's parent associations and petition to change the school's homework policy to a more reasonable amount. The goal here is to help children achieve a balance between school work and home life. Your child will benefit more from fun family activities instead.[12] There is no harm in after-school activities, especially if your child enjoys them. However, the rest of the time should be spent interacting and playing with family and friends, doing things they enjoy.

4: Be a Good Role Model

Parents influence their children in meaningful ways by how they live their lives, even when no one else is looking. Kids learn how to solve problems and critically think about the world around them, in part, by observing their parents. Small children are like sponges, and they will absorb and mimic their parents' behaviors as well as their diet and lifestyle habits. If you want your child to one day be an honest, upstanding citizen who is caring and compassionate, you need to be that yourself.[13]

5: Hang Out with Your Child

The main rule of being a good parent is fostering a secure and warm attachment with your kids; that way they know their needs will be met and that they'll have a place to go to when they need comfort. It is critical for their emotional development to spend regular time with your kids and ask them open-ended questions about themselves and about how they see the world. Actively listen to their responses; you will learn all kinds of things that make your child unique.[14]

As your children grow, their needs will change. They will need more independence and a feeling of control. After all, they are turning into self-sufficient human beings. You need to gradually loosen the reins and give them opportunities to make mistakes and learn from them.

6: Show Your Child More Respect

Showing respect means that you listen to your children and take them seriously, which conveys to them that what they think and feel is important to you and has merit. This teaches them self-respect. Believing in and guiding your kids to get back on their feet after a setback will help them believe in themselves and make them more resilient as adults.[15,16] Teaching children that failure is not a bad thing is a great life skill that will allow them to make smart decisions and learn from life's ups and downs.

7: Praise the Behavior, Not the Child

When it comes to performance, praise the behavior you desire. Praise children for their hard work and be task specific[17] instead of calling them smart. When you label children as "smart," their ego gets tied to their performance and makes them unwilling to take on challenges because of the fear of failure. They believe their achievements come from their innate abilities,[18] and any failure would destroy their ego. When children are praised for being hard working, determined, and self-disciplined, they are usually more willing to face challenges with hard work and their grades reflect their efforts. The same concept can be applied to disruptive behaviors. By correcting their actions and placing appropriate consequences that fit the misbehavior, you are not hurting their self-worth but giving them the opportunity to learn from and adjust their behavior. For example, if your child has a curfew and came home late one night, a fitting consequence might be to come home early the next time.[19]

8: The Importance of Hugs

Hug your children every day, several times a day, and hold them with your loving embrace until they squirm and want to get out. Studies have shown that hugging and interacting with a nurturing touch helps children regulate their emotions. It also lowers the stress hormone cortisol and boosts the immune system.[20]

The loving relationship formed between you and your children and your interactions with them provide the foundation for their higher thinking skills as well. Children are resilient in every way. They heal faster, they absorb information faster, and, when they are small, they will mimic their parents like a monkey. In essence, they are thermometers for what is going on in the household. Their behavior will be a direct result of the emotional climate of the home. Make sure to keep an emotionally stable and happy environment in the house.

9: Make Music a Part of Your Child's Life

Studies have shown that listening to music can lower stress levels[21] and engage the areas of the brain involved in paying attention.[22] A slower rhythm and music from stringed instruments, drums, and flutes can be effective at creating a relaxation response. Sounds of nature can also be relaxing when paired with easy-listening music. The most important factor is that you have to like the music being played. Forcing yourself to listen to relaxing music that irritates you will create tension, not stress reduction.[23]

Playing a musical instrument has an added effect on the brain's spatial-temporal thinking, which may help in solving abstract math.[24] Learning to play an instrument is not for everyone, and parents should not put the added pressure on their children unnecessarily. However, if your girl, for example, is showing an aptitude for music and enjoys it, let her try different instruments until she finds what she likes, and encourage her to stick with it.

10: Encourage Your Kids to Go Out and Play

Playing outside is important, especially now more than ever, with children glued to their smart devices and different technologies all day long. Physical exercise makes your child smart, with improvements in attention and working memory.[25] Vigorous physical activity not only makes your child strong and fit, but it also increases blood flow and glucose to the brain, which can improve their concentration. It also helps create new neural connections in their brains. Exercise will also help children manage stress and anxiety more effectively and set them up for a lifelong trajectory for good health. It is important that they get out every day and have moderate physical activities for at least thirty minutes to see any of these benefits.[26]

Let your kids play outside in the dirt; it will help train and modulate their immune systems and reduce the odds of them developing autoimmune conditions such as asthma or eczema.[27] But make sure the environment your child plays in is not contaminated with anything, such as animal feces, that could contain parasites. If your child is already immune compromised, be more cautious. Minimize his or her exposure to unknown pathogens by letting them play in a more controlled setting.

11: Nutrition Is Crucial for Their Development

Children's young, growing bodies are more sensitive to small changes in their diet. Make sure they get good, wholesome food, with most of their calories coming from home-cooked foods made with single-ingredient products such as meats, vegetables, grains, and spices. Include a rainbow of colors in the fruits and vegetables they consume. Multiple colors on their plate may make the food more appealing to children and provide a range of beneficial micronutrients. Giving them fast foods such as burgers and pizzas or premade meals such as boxed mac and cheese once in a while should be okay as long as they eat healthy most of the time.

It can take several exposures for children to accept the taste of a food they are not fond of, so don't give up too soon. Pairing a new, unfamiliar food with an old favorite will trick their picky taste buds into accepting it.

12: Children Grow in Their Sleep

If you want your children to grow to their full potential, make sure they get the proper amount of sleep. Even a small sleep deficit seems to have negative health effects, such as severe headaches and depression.[28] Babies under one year can sleep up to seventeen hours a day. From one to five years of age, twelve hours seems sufficient, and from six to seventeen years of age, ten hours is adequate.[29] These are only estimates extrapolated from a narrower range of recommendations by the National Sleep Foundation. Your child may sleep a little more or less than this, and that is normal. Keep in mind that overtired children can become hyperactive. If this is the case, they generally don't slow down, but they speed up until they crash. Keeping consistent, relaxing bedtime routines will be helpful, and just like with adults, keeping the bedroom cool, dark, and quiet will be conducive to proper sleeping.

Daytime naps can help kids from becoming overtired, which can affect their moods and make it harder for them to fall asleep at night. How much children nap is individualized and depends on their needs. If your child is showing signs of hyperactivity or aggression, having trouble focusing, or getting cranky or irritable in the late afternoon, he or she may be sleep deprived and could benefit from napping during the day.[30]

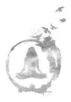

RULES FOR *Healthy Aging*

It may seem pointless for an eighty-year-old to one day start living a healthy life after a lifetime of self-indulgence and damaging behaviors, but there may still be hope. I give this extreme example because I know how forgiving our bodies can be and how amazing it is at healing itself. When we talk about healthy aging, it is not only about living a longer life but also about living a higher-quality life for the remainder of your years—living life to its fullest each day, no matter how old you are.

As a society, we value looking young and spend an exorbitant amount of resources at preserving our youth, but that sets a false notion in the minds of millions that youth is all there is, and once lost, there is only decay and lifelessness. I am here to dispel this myth. Age is just a number. I have seen sixty-year-olds who can run circles around thirty-year-olds with how vibrant and fulfilling their lives are. Granted, for the time being, no one can win the war against mortality, and change is inevitable as we age, but how we accept this change is of paramount importance.

For the average person, as we age, our bodies start to slow down and deteriorate. Aches and pains become our everyday companions and chronic diseases become our milestones. But what if this is not inevitable? Can we live a healthy life right up to the end? The answer is yes, but it also depends on your expectations. Do you want to get younger every day, or do you want to maintain good health? No one has found the fountain of youth, so let's focus on the more achievable latter. There is a reason I left this chapter for the end. Everything we have discussed up until this point will in some way contribute to healthy aging. Specifically, focusing on a diet rich in plant matter and omega-3-rich fish, getting high-quality sleep, exercising, and keeping your stress levels checked are vital to healthy aging. Certain things will also shorten your life span, such as smoking, drinking excessively, and being sedentary.[1,2] It's always a balancing act. There will be periods in your life where you may succumb to unhealthy behavior, such as binge drinking or eating junk food, and that is just part of life. However, being aware of the consequences and taking steps to improve your lifestyle habits will be to your benefit in the long run.

Let's explore strategies that may help you age gracefully.

1: Antioxidants, the Misunderstood Hero

Our body's metabolic processes naturally produce free radicals or reactive oxygen species (ROS). If gone unchecked, these molecules can strip electrons from nearby molecules, leading to a chain reaction of oxidative damage. This may be the underlying reason for many degenerative changes we see with aging.[3] Fortunately, there are natural antioxidant mechanisms within the body that actively neutralize these free radicals. However, with age, their abilities diminish and dietary antioxidants take precedence. These come in the form of vitamins and phytochemicals naturally occurring in plant life.

Certain foods may provide a higher antioxidant value, and the oxygen radical absorbance capacity (ORAC) is one way of identifying these foods. It assigns higher scores to fruits, vegetables, and spices that provide the most antioxidant capacity, as measured in a test tube.[4] How well this translates to real-life effects within a human body is still debatable and should be taken with a grain of salt. Don't base your decisions solely on how high the ORAC rating is; there are many biochemical means for reducing cellular damage, most of which are poorly understood. However, it does show us that there is some merit in looking at the patterns these values show us and going for brightly colored produce, which usually score high. The pigments in these plants provide us with protective benefits, so the goal for you should be to get a variety of colors (green, yellow, red, orange, and purple) in your veggies and fruits.

- One of the easiest things you can do is to start drinking two to three cups of green tea daily. The polyphenol EGCG (epigallocatechin gallate) found in green tea is an effective antioxidant and seems to provide antiaging skin protection.[5,6]
- Eat wild berries, such as blueberries, bilberries, strawberries, elderberries, and raspberries, regularly whenever they are in season, or get them frozen if out of season. The anthocyanins found in berries provide benefits in reducing age-associated oxidative stress.[7,8]
- Other foods to incorporate into your diet would be cruciferous vegetables, such as broccoli, brussels sprouts, and cauliflower, and their dark-green varieties, such as kale and collards. These contain a range of organosulfur compounds, which are great at reducing the oxidant load.[9]
- Avocados, beets, pomegranates, sweet potatoes, and tomatoes are all highly nutritious and beneficial foods worth including regularly in a well-rounded diet to get that extra boost of antioxidants. The trick with tomatoes is to eat them cooked to maximize the lycopene absorption and to go for the reddest tomatoes you can find.
- Use a variety of spices in cooking your food, especially turmeric, which has received a lot of attention in recent years for its antioxidant

and anti-inflammatory effects. The unknown trick with using turmeric is to add a pinch of black pepper to increase its bioavailability by 2,000 percent.[10]

- Just because certain foods are high in antioxidants does not mean you should eat large quantities of such foods in exclusion of others. The body always plays with a delicate balance of processes, and a balance of antioxidants and prooxidants must be maintained. Some folks think that just because a little bit of something is good, then a lot of it must be better, but that is not the case here. Always strive for balance. For example, if you had burgers and fries for lunch, aim to have an avocado and a nice salad for dinner. This is not giving you permission to eat more unhealthy food but to know that when you do, you should try to balance it with healthier foods.

- Try to get your antioxidants from food sources as much as you can and don't rely on supplements to fill in the gap. Taking large doses of antioxidant supplements may do more harm than good if not done properly under professional guidance, especially if you have preexisting medical conditions.

2: Mitochondria, the Powerhouse

Most of the energy you produce in your body comes from tiny organelles in your cells called mitochondria. It has been postulated that aging and most chronic degenerative conditions come about because of breakdown or dysfunction in our mitochondria.[11] It would seem logical that by improving our mitochondria's function, we can essentially improve our health and prolong our lives. Oversupply of calories and inactivity seem to be at the root of most chronic diseases.[12] In animal experiments, rats fed a diet high in fructose developed significant damage to the mitochondria in their liver, with an inability to repair and renew them.[13] So what can we do to preserve our mitochondrial health? We have been doing so all along throughout this book, but to emphasize healthy aging strategies, make sure to implement the following:

- Eat a diet rich in fruits and vegetables, with reduced calories coming from processed carbs and sugars. Cut your calorie intake slightly by removing high-carb foods from your diet and rely more on getting your carbs from vegetables that are nutrient packed.
- Move often and exercise regularly, doing both endurance and resistance-based exercises to make your mitochondria multiply and be more efficient.[14]
- Reduce your exposure to tobacco smoke and air pollution in general to help preserve your mitochondria.[15]

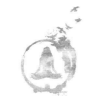

Conclusion

Well done! That was a lot of information to process in a short while. My advice would be to come back to this book regularly and take from it what you need. You can prioritize based on what you need most to optimize your health. Some people might benefit from ensuring they get higher-quality sleep. Others might benefit from improving their diet, and almost everyone could benefit from managing their stress effectively. There is no rush. Take as much time as you need. In time, you will have mastered all the rules to live a balanced and healthy life.

I will emphasize some key points to drive home the essence of this book.

When it comes to leading a healthy life, don't compare yourself to others. We are constantly bombarded with images of slim or muscular individuals and influenced into thinking that one must be a certain size or shape to be healthy. That is far from the truth. You can be overweight and be healthy. On the flip side, you can be slim and be unhealthy. Health takes into account multiple factors, and focusing just on looks may not be in your best interest. Instead, focus on how you feel, how much energy you have throughout the day, how sharp your mind is, or how well you sleep. Get your blood work done to make sure everything is okay. Get your bases covered from following all the rules in this book.

A famous quote attributed to Hippocrates says, "Let food be thy medicine and medicine be thy food." Even in the early stages of modern medicines, it was realized that food plays an important role in keeping people healthy and that eating right could be considered medicinal.

Realize the power of having wholesome, good-quality food. Most diseases happen as a result of an imbalance within us, and their cause usually originates in the gut, which is why I have placed such a strong emphasis on making what you put into your body a priority. However, it doesn't mean you should ignore other areas of your health. You can eat the best-quality food in the world, but if you lead a stressful life and don't sleep well, your health will undoubtedly suffer.

Realize the connection of mind and body. The brain sits on top of the body because it's in charge. Just as individuals do their best to give their bodies good-quality food, the mind also needs good-quality food in the form of peaceful thoughts. Our thoughts are extremely powerful in the way they influence our health. Negative thoughts will drain your life force. Be aware of your thoughts by being more mindful through meditation and introspection. By stopping the train of negative thoughts and bringing the focus back into your body, there will be a reduction in their frequency and more peace of mind.

Optimal health happens as a result of a beautiful amalgam of biological and psychological processes, working in harmony for the benefit of one organism: you. All you need to do is listen to the clues from within, provide good sustenance and peace of mind, and get out of the way and let your body do its thing. This is the simplicity in the complexity of who we are as human beings. It's always a balancing act. Nobody gets it right all the time. All you can do is try your best.

I hope you have found this book to be of value for you and your family. Bringing hope and knowledge into this world is my passion, and I look forward to providing you with many more books in the coming years. Thank you.

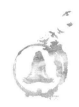

References

Intro

1: Cohen S, Janicki-Deverts D, Doyle WJ, et al. Chronic stress, glucocorticoid receptor resistance, inflammation, and disease risk. *Proc. Natl. Acad. Sci. U.S.A.* 2012;109(16):5995–5999.

Air

1: Peel RG, et al. Seasonal variation in diurnal atmospheric grass pollen concentration profiles. *Biogeosciences.* 2014;11:821–832.

2: U.S. Census Bureau, 2012–2016, American Community Survey 5-year estimates. Mean travel time to work (minutes).

3: Nowak DJ, et al. Oxygen production by urban trees. *Arboriculture & Urban Forestry.* 2007;33(3):220–226.

4: Wolverton BC, et al. A study of interior landscape plants for indoor air pollution abatement: an interim report. NASA. September 1989.

5: Tang YY, Tang R, Posner MI. Brief meditation training induces smoking reduction. *Proc Natl Acad Sci U S A.* 2013 Aug 20;110(34):13971–13975.

6: Bennett MP, Zeller JM, Rosenberg L, McCann J. The effect of mirthful laughter on stress and natural killer cell activity. *Altern Ther Health Med.* 2003 Mar–Apr;9(2):38–45.

7: Arundel AV, Sterling EM, Biggin JH, Sterling TD. Indirect health effects of relative humidity in indoor environments. *Environmental Health Perspectives.* 1986;65:351–361.

Water

1: Chumlea WC, Guo SS, Zeller CM, Reo NV, Siervogel RM. Total body water data for white adults 18 to 64 years of age: The Fels Longitudinal Study. *Kidney International.* 1999;56(1):244–252.

2: Goodman AB, Blanck HM, Sherry B, Park S, Nebeling L, Yaroch AL. Behaviors and attitudes associated with low drinking water intake among US adults, food attitudes and behaviors survey, 2007. *Prev Chronic Dis.* 2013;10:120248.

3: Saker P, Farrell MJ, Egan GF, McKinley MJ, Denton DA. Overdrinking, swallowing inhibition, and regional brain responses prior to swallowing. *Proc Natl Acad Sci U S A.* October 6, 2016;113(43):12274–12279.

4: Szaro J, Hernandez P, Singh A, Fagan JM. Warning: BPA Toxicity. Don't Heat Food with "Plastic." A Proposal for Labeling in Grocery Stores.

5: Kinch CD, Ibhazehiebo K, Jeong J-H, Habibi HR, Kurrasch DM. Low-dose exposure to bisphenol A and replacement bisphenol S induces precocious hypothalamic neurogenesis in embryonic zebrafish. *Proc Natl Acad Sci U S A.* 2015;112(5):1475–1480.

6: http://nutritiondata.self.com. Searched under tools; nutrient search tool; find foods that are highest in water. Similar procedure used for subsequent searches.

7: Institute of Medicine. Dietary reference intake for water, potassium, sodium, chloride and sulfate. *The National Academic Press.* Washington, 2004.

8: Popkin BM, D'Anci KE, Rosenberg IH. Water, hydration and health. *Nutrition Reviews.* 2010;68(8):439-458.

9: Roberts J, Freeman J. Hydrotherapy management of low back pain: a quality improvement project. *Aust J Physiother.* 1995;41(3):205-208.

10: Mooventhan A, Nivethitha L. Scientific evidence-based effects of hydrotherapy on various systems of the body. *North American Journal of Medical Sciences.* 2014;6(5):199-209.

11: https://www.scientificamerican.com/article/supercharging-brown-fat-to-battle-obesity. Accessed June 20, 2018.

12: Boyle W, Saine A. "Lectures in Naturopathic Hydrotherapy." Eclectic Medical Publications. Sandy, Oregon, 1988.

13: Kai Olson-Sawyer, "Beef has a big water footprint. Here's why." Grace Communications Foundation, March 14, 2017. http://www.gracelinks.org/blog/7858. Accessed June 20, 2018.

14: Kai Olson-Sawyer, "Beef: The 'King' of the Big Water Footprints." Grace Communications Foundation, August 1, 2011. http://www.gracelinks.org/blog/1143/beef-the-king-of-the-big-water-footprints. Accessed June 20, 2018.

15: "Product Gallery." Water Footprint Network. http://waterfootprint.org/en/resources/interactive-tools/product-gallery. Accessed June 20, 2018.

Food

1: Micha R, Wallace SK, Mozaffarian D. Red and processed meat consumption and risk of incident coronary heart disease, stroke, and diabetes mellitus: a systematic review and meta-analysis. *Circulation.* 2010 Jun 1;121(21):2271-2283.

2: Larsson SC, Bergkvist L, Wolk A. Processed meat consumption, dietary nitrosamines and stomach cancer risk in a cohort of Swedish women. *Int J Cancer.* 2006 Aug 15;119(4):915-919.

3: Hamilton MC, Hites RA, Schwager SJ, Foran JA, Knuth BA, Carpenter DO. Lipid composition and contaminants in farmed and wild salmon. *Environ Sci Technol.* 2005 Nov 15;39(22):8622-8629.

4: Sabaté J. The contribution of vegetarian diets to health and disease: a paradigm shift? *The American Journal of Clinical Nutrition*, 2003; 78(3):502S-507S.

5: https://www.ewg.org/foodnews/dirty-dozen.php. Accessed June 22, 2018.

6: Ibid.

7: https://www.ucsusa.org/food-agriculture/advance-sustainable-agriculture/what-is-sustainable-agriculture. Accessed June 22, 2018.

8: http://rodaleinstitute.org/why-local-food-is-better-for-you. Accessed June 22, 2018.

9: Titanium Dioxide Classified as Possibly Carcinogenic to Humans. Retrieved May 21, 2018, from Canadian Centre for Occupational Health and Safety.

10: Tobacman JK. Review of harmful gastrointestinal effects of carrageenan in animal experiments. *Environmental Health Perspectives.* 2001;109(10):983-994.

11: Borthakur A, Bhattacharyya S, Anbazhagan AN, Kumar A, Dudeja PK, Tobacman JK. Prolongation of carrageenan-induced inflammation in human colonic epithelial cells by activation of an NFκB-BCL10 loop. *Biochim Biophys Acta.* 2012 Aug;1822(8):1300-1307.

12: Pugazhendhi D, Pope GS, Darbre PD. Oestrogenic activity of p-hydroxybenzoic acid (common metabolite of paraben esters) and methylparaben in human breast cancer cell lines. *J Appl Toxicol.* 2005 Jul-Aug;25(4):301-309.

13: Tipton KD, Elliott TA, Cree MG, Aarsland AA, Sanford AP, Wolfe RR. Stimulation of net muscle protein synthesis by whey protein ingestion before and after exercise. *American Journal of Physiology-Endocrinology and Metabolism.* 2007;292:1,E71–E76.

14: Peter S, Chopra S, Jacob JJ. A fish a day keeps the cardiologist away! A review of the effect of omega-3 fatty acids in the cardiovascular system. *Indian Journal of Endocrinology and Metabolism.* 2013;17(3):422–429.

15: Raji CA, Erickson KI, Lopez OL, Kuller LH, Gach HM, Thompson PM, Riverol M, Becker JT. Regular fish consumption and age-related brain gray matter loss. *Am J Prev Med.* 2014 Oct;47(4):444–451.

16: http://nutritiondata.self.com. Searched under tools; nutrient search tool; foods highest in total omega-3 fatty acids. Accessed April 18, 2018.

17: Peter S, Chopra S, Jacob JJ. A fish a day keeps the cardiologist away! A review of the effect of omega-3 fatty acids in the cardiovascular system. *Indian Journal of Endocrinology and Metabolism.* 2013;17(3):422–429.

18: Lee JG, Kim SY, Moon JS, Kim SH, Kang DH, Yoon HJ. Effects of grilling procedures on levels of polycyclic aromatic hydrocarbons in grilled meats. *Food Chem.* 2016 May 15;199:632–638.

19: White AJ, Bradshaw PT, Herring AH, Teitelbaum SL, Beyea J, Stellman SD, Steck SE, Mordukhovich I, Eng SM, Engel LS, Conway K, Hatch M, Neugut AI, Santella RM, Gammon MD. Exposure to multiple sources of polycyclic aromatic hydrocarbons and breast cancer incidence. *Environ Int.* 2016 Apr-May;89-90:185–192.

20: Lee JG, Kim SY, Moon JS, Kim SH, Kang DH, Yoon HJ. Effects of grilling procedures on levels of polycyclic aromatic hydrocarbons in grilled meats. *Food Chem.* 2016 May 15;199:632–638.

21: Corn Refiners Association. Corn Oil. 5th ed. 2006.

22: *Sherwood L, Willey J, Woolverton C. Prescott's Microbiology.* 9th ed. New York: McGraw Hill; 2013:713–721.

23: *Quigley EM.* Gut bacteria in health and disease. *Gastroenterol Hepatol.* New York: 2013;9:560–569.

24: Parvez S, Malik KA, Ah Kang S, Kim H-Y. Probiotics and their fermented food products are beneficial for health. *Journal of Applied Microbiology.* 2006;100(6):1171–1185.

25: Rao AV, Bested AC, Beaulne TM, Katzman MA, Iorio C, Berardi JM, Logan AC. A randomized, double-blind, placebo-controlled pilot study of a probiotic in emotional symptoms of chronic fatigue syndrome. *Gut Pathogens.* 2009;1:6.

26: Institute for Agriculture and Trade Policy. Much High Fructose Corn Syrup Contaminated with Mercury, New Study Finds. Jan. 25, 2009.

27: Kelly JR, Kennedy PJ, Cryan JF, Dinan TG, Clarke G, Hyland NP. Breaking down the barriers: the gut microbiome, intestinal permeability and stress-related psychiatric disorders. *Frontiers in Cellular Neuroscience.* 2015;9:392.

Sleep

1: Patel SR, Hu FB. Short sleep duration and weight gain: a systematic review. *Obesity.* 2008;16:643–653.

2: Leproult R, Van Cauter E. Role of sleep and sleep loss in hormonal release and metabolism. *Endocr Dev.* 2010;17:11–21.

3: Taheri S, Lin L, Austin D, Young T, Mignot E. Short sleep duration is associated with reduced leptin, elevated ghrelin, and increased body mass index. *PLoS Med.* 2004 Dec;1(3):e62.

4: Cappuccio FP(1), Cooper D, D'Elia L, Strazzullo P, Miller MA. Sleep duration predicts cardiovascular outcomes: a systematic review and meta-analysis of prospective studies. *Eur Heart J.* 2011 Jun;32(12):1484–1492.

5: Irwin M, McClintick J, Costlow C, Fortner M, White J, Gillin JC. Partial night sleep deprivation reduces natural killer and cellular immune responses in humans. *FASEB J.* 1996 Apr;10(5):643–653.

6: Hayley AC, Williams LJ, Venugopal K, Kennedy GA, Berk M, Pasco JA. The relationships between insomnia, sleep apnoea and depression: findings from the American National Health and Nutrition Examination Survey, 2005-2008. *Aust N Z J Psychiatry.* 2015 Feb;49(2):156–170.

7: Hirshkowitz M, et al. National Sleep Foundation's sleep time duration recommendations: methodology and results summary. Sleep Health: *Journal of the National Sleep Foundation.* 2015;1(1):40–43.

8: Gooley JJ, Chamberlain K, Smith KA, et al. Exposure to room light before bedtime suppresses melatonin onset and shortens melatonin duration in humans. *The Journal of Clinical Endocrinology and Metabolism.* 2011;96(3):E463–E472.

9: Zhao J, Tian Y, Nie J, Xu J, Liu D. Red light and the sleep quality and endurance performance of Chinese female basketball players. *Journal of Athletic Training.* 2012;47(6):673–678.

10: Cagnacci A. Influences of melatonin on human circadian rhythms. *Chronobiol Int.* 1997 Mar;14(2):205–20.

11: https://wellwithin.net/energymedicinetopics/adrenal-fatigue. Accessed June 23, 2018.

12: Brainard GC, et al. Action spectrum for melatonin regulation in humans: evidence for a novel circadian photoreceptor. *J Neurosci.* 2001;21:6405–6412.

13: Matheson A, O'Brien L, Reid JA. The impact of shiftwork on health: a literature review. *J Clin Nurs.* 2014;23(23-24):3309–3320.

14: McMillan DE, Fallis WM. Benefits of napping on night shifts. *Nursing Times.* 2011 Nov 8-14;107(44):12–13.

15: Mednick SC, Cai DJ, Kanady J, Drummond SPA. Comparing the benefits of caffeine, naps and placebo on verbal, motor and perceptual memory. *Behavioural Brain Research.* 2008;193(1):79–86.

16: http://thebreathproject.org/how-to-relieve-stress/progressive-muscle-relaxation. Accessed June 24, 2018.

17: https://www.anxietybc.com/adults/how-do-progressive-muscle-relaxation. Accessed June 24, 2018

18: Kredlow MA, Capozzoli MC, Hearon BA, Calkins AW, Otto MW. The effects of physical activity on sleep: a meta-analytic review. *J Behav Med.* 2015 Jun;38(3):427–449.

19: Youngstedt SD, O'Connor PJ, Dishman RK. The effects of acute exercise on sleep: a quantitative synthesis. *Sleep.* 1997;20(3):203–214.

Exercise

1: Warburton DER, Nicol CW, Bredin SSD. Health benefits of physical activity: the evidence. *CMAJ.* March 14, 2006;174(6):801–809.

2: Reiner M, Niermann C, Jekauc D, Woll A. Long-term health benefits of physical activity: a systematic review of longitudinal studies. *BMC Public Health.* 2013;13(813).

3: Shiraev T, Barclay G. Evidence based exercise: clinical benefits of high intensity interval training. *Australian Family Physician.* 2012;41(12): 960–962.

4: Herbert RD, Gabriel M. Effects of stretching before and after exercising on muscle soreness and risk of injury: systematic review. *BMJ.* 2002; 325:468.

5: Cipriani D, Abel B, Pirrwitz D. A comparison of two stretching protocols on hip range of motion: implications for total daily stretch duration. *J Strength Cond Res.* 2003 May;17(2):274–278.

6: Rackow P, Scholz U, Hornung R. Received social support and exercising: an intervention study to test the enabling hypothesis. *British Journal of Health Psychology.* 2015;20(4):763.

7: Ibid.

8: Blumenthal JA, Emery CF, Madden DJ, George LK, Coleman RE, Riddle MW, McKee DC, Reasoner J, Williams RS. Cardiovascular and behavioral effects of aerobic exercise training in healthy older men and women. *Journal of Gerontology.* 1989;44(5):M147–M157.

9: Smith PJ, Blumenthal JA, Hoffman BM, et al. Aerobic exercise and neurocognitive performance: a meta-analytic review of randomized controlled trials. *Psychosomatic Medicine.* 2010;72(3):239–252.

10: Lee S, Bacha F, Hannon T, Kuk JL, Boesch C, Arslanian S. Effects of aerobic versus resistance exercise without caloric restriction on abdominal fat, intrahepatic lipid, and insulin sensitivity in obese adolescent boys. *Diabetes.* Nov 2012;6(11):2787–2795.

11: Koopman R, Manders RJ, Zorenc AH, Hul GB, Kuipers H, Keizer HA, van Loon LJ. A single session of resistance exercise enhances insulin sensitivity for at least 24 h in healthy men. *Eur J Appl Physiol.* 2005 May;94(1–2):180–187.

12: Phillips SM. Dietary protein requirements and adaptive advantages in athletes. *Br J Nutr.* 2012 Aug;108 Suppl 2:S158–167.

13: Shimomura Y, Yamamoto Y, Bajotto G, Sato J, Murakami T, Shimomura N, Kobayashi H, Mawatari K. Nutraceutical effects of branched-chain amino acids on skeletal muscle. *J Nutr.* 2006 Feb;136(2):529S–532S.

14: Casey A, Greenhaff PL. Does dietary creatine supplementation play a role in skeletal muscle metabolism and performance? *The American Journal of Clinical Nutrition.* 2000 August;72(2):607S–617S.

15: Wilmot EG, Edwardson CL, Achana FA, Davies MJ, Gorely T, Gray LJ, Khunti K, Yates T, Biddle SJ. Sedentary time in adults and the association with diabetes, cardiovascular disease and death: systematic review and meta-analysis. *Diabetologia.* 2012 Nov;55(11):2895–2905.

16: Van der Ploeg HP, Chey T, Korda RJ, Banks E, Bauman A. Sitting time and all-cause mortality risk in 222 497 Australian adults. *Arch Intern Med.* 2012 Mar 26;172(6):494–500.

17: Wilmot EG, Edwardson CL, Achana FA, Davies MJ, Gorely T, Gray LJ, Khunti K, Yates T, Biddle SJ. Sedentary time in adults and the association with diabetes, cardiovascular disease and death: systematic review and meta-analysis. *Diabetologia.* 2012 Nov;55(11):2895–2905.

Stress

1: D'Amico D, Libro G, Prudenzano MP, et al. Stress and chronic headache. *The Journal of Headache and Pain.* 2000;1(Suppl 1):S49–S52.

2: Graham NM, Douglas RM, Ryan P. Stress and acute respiratory infection. *Am J Epidemiol.* 1986 Sep;124(3):389–401.

3: Van Uum SH, Sauvé B, Fraser LA, Morley-Forster P, Paul TL, Koren G. Elevated content of cortisol in hair of patients with severe chronic pain: a novel biomarker for stress. *Stress.* 2008 Nov;11(6):483–488.

4: Kocalevent RD, Hinz A, Brähler E, Klapp BF. Determinants of fatigue and stress. *BMC Res Notes.* 2011 Jul 20;4:238.

5: Hertig VL, Cain KC, Jarrett ME, Burr RL, Heitkemper MM. Daily stress and gastrointestinal symptoms in women with irritable bowel syndrome. *Nurs Res.* 2007 Nov-Dec;56(6):399–406.

6: Sangi-Haghpeykar H, Ambani DS, Carson SA. Stress, workload, sexual well-being and quality of life among physician residents in training. *Int J Clin Pract.* 2009 Mar;63(3):462–467.

7: Hammen C, Kim EY, Eberhart NK, Brennan PA. Chronic and acute stress and the prediction of major depression in women. *Depress Anxiety.* 2009;26(8):718–723.

8: Irigaray P, Newby JA, Clapp R, Hardell L, Howard V, Montagnier L, Epstein S, Belpomme D. Lifestyle-related factors and environmental agents causing cancer: an overview. *Biomed Pharmacother.* 2007 Dec;61(10):640–658.

9: Ames BN. Identifying environmental chemicals causing mutations and cancer. *Science.* 1979 May 11;204(4393):587–593.

10: Heath CW Jr. Electromagnetic field exposure and cancer: a review of epidemiologic evidence. *CA Cancer J Clin.* 1996 Jan-Feb;46(1):29–44.

11: Gandhi OP, Morgan LL, de Salles AA, Han YY, Herberman RB, Davis DL. Exposure limits: the underestimation of absorbed cell phone radiation, especially in children. *Electromagn Biol Med.* 2012 Mar;31(1):34–51.

12: Christ A, Gosselin MC, Christopoulou M, Kühn S, Kuster N. Age-dependent tissue-specific exposure of cell phone users. *Phys Med Biol.* 2010 Apr 7;55(7):1767–1783.

13: Goyal M, Singh S, Sibinga EM, Gould NF, Rowland-Seymour A, Sharma R, Berger Z, Sleicher D, Maron DD, Shihab HM, Ranasinghe PD, Linn S, Saha S, Bass EB, Haythornthwaite JA. Meditation programs for psychological stress and well-being: a systematic review and meta-analysis. *JAMA Intern Med.* 2014 Mar;174(3):357–368.

14: Chen KW, Berger CC, Manheimer E, Forde D, Magidson J, Dachman L, Lejuez CW. Meditative therapies for reducing anxiety: a systematic review and meta-analysis of randomized controlled trials. *Depress Anxiety.* 2012 Jul;29(7):545–562.

15: Jain FA, Walsh RN, Eisendrath SJ, Christensen S, Rael Cahn B. Critical analysis of the efficacy of meditation therapies for acute and subacute phase treatment of depressive disorders: a systematic review. *Psychosomatics.* 2015 Mar-Apr;56(2):140–152.

16: Rosenkranz MA, Davidson RJ, Maccoon DG, Sheridan JF, Kalin NH, Lutz A. A comparison of mindfulness-based stress reduction and an active control in modulation of neurogenic inflammation. *Brain Behav Immun.* 2013 Jan;27(1):174–184.

17: Martires J, Zeidler M. The value of mindfulness meditation in the treatment of insomnia. *Curr Opin Pulm Med.* 2015 Nov;21(6):547–552.

18: Goyal M, Singh S, Sibinga EM, Gould NF, Rowland-Seymour A, Sharma R, Berger Z, Sleicher D, Maron DD, Shihab HM, Ranasinghe PD, Linn S, Saha S, Bass EB, Haythornthwaite JA. Meditation programs for psychological stress and well-being: a systematic review and meta-analysis. *JAMA Intern Med.* 2014 Mar;174(3):357–368.

19: Ricard M, Lutz A, Davidson RJ. Mind of the meditator. November 2014. ScientificAmerican.com.

20: Berman MG, Kross E, Krpan KM, et al. Interacting with nature improves cognition and affect for individuals with depression. *Journal of Affective Disorders.* 2012;140(3):300–305.

21: Bratman GN, Daily GC, Levy BJ, Gross JJ. The benefits of nature experience: improved affect and cognition. *Landscape and Urban Planning.* 2015;138:41–50.

22: Tsunetsugu Y, Park BJ, Miyazaki Y. Trends in research related to "Shinrin-yoku" (taking in the forest atmosphere or forest bathing) in Japan. *Environ Health Prev Med.* 2010;15:27–37.

Relationships

1: Cohen S. Social relationships and health. *Am Psychol.* 2004 Nov;59(8):676–684.

2: Post SG. Altruism, happiness, and health: it's good to be good. *Int J BehavMed.* 2005;12(2):66–77.

3: Weisberg YJ, DeYoung CG, Hirsh JB. Gender differences in personality across the ten aspects of the big five. *Frontiers in Psychology.* 2011;2:178.

4: Del Giudice M, Booth T, Irwing P. *The Distance Between Mars and Venus: Measuring Global Sex Differences in Personality.* Avenanti A, ed. *PLoS ONE.* 2012;7(1):e29265.

5: Gove WR, Hughes M, Style CB. Does marriage have positive effects on the psychological well-being of the individual? *J Health Soc Behav.* 1983 Jun;24(2):122–131.

6: Powell LH, Shahabi L, Thoresen CE. Religion and spirituality: linkages to physical health. *Am Psychol.* 2003 Jan;58(1):36–52.

7: Brown DR, Gary LE. Religious involvement and health status among African-American males. *Journal of the National Medical Association.* 1994;86(11):825–831.

8: Watkins PC, Woodward K, Stone T, Kolts RL. Gratitude and happiness: development of a measure of gratitude, and relationships with subjective well-being. *Social Behavior and Personality: An International Journal.* 2003;31(5):431–451.

Mind

1: Sánchez-Villegas A, Toledo E, de Irala J, Ruiz-Canela M, Pla-Vidal J, Martínez-González MA. Fast-food and commercial baked goods consumption and the risk of depression. *Public Health Nutr.* 2012 Mar;15(3):424–432.

2: Hartshorne JK, Germine LT. When does cognitive functioning peak? The asynchronous rise and fall of different cognitive abilities across the life span. *Psychol Sci.* 2015 Apr;26(4):433–443.

3: Daily crosswords linked to sharper brain in later life. http://www.exeter.ac.uk/news/featurednews/title_595009_en.html. Accessed May 26, 2018.

4: Cahill L, McGaugh JL. A novel demonstration of enhanced memory associated with emotional arousal. *Conscious Cogn.* 1995 Dec;4(4):410–421.

5: Kok BE, Coffey KA, Cohn MA, Catalino LI, Vacharkulksemsuk T, Algoe SB, Brantley M, Fredrickson BL. How positive emotions build physical health: perceived positive social connections account for the upward spiral between positive emotions and vagal tone. *Psychol Sci.* 2013 Jul 1;24(7):1123–1132.

Detox

1: https://biochemistrymedicine.wordpress.com/2014/06/28/why-is-ammonia-toxic-to-the-body. Accessed June 25, 2018.

2: https://www.med.uio.no/imb/english/research/news-and-events/news/2014/when-ammonia-becomes-toxic.html. Accessed June 25, 2018.

3: https://medlineplus.gov/ency/article/000281.htm. Accessed June 25, 2018.

4: https://www.cdc.gov/alcohol/fact-sheets/moderate-drinking.htm. Accessed June 25, 2018.

5: El-Zayadi A-R. Heavy smoking and liver. *World Journal of Gastroenterology: WJG.* 2006;12(38):6098–6101.

6: https://www.cdc.gov/tobacco/data_statistics/fact_sheets/health_effects/effects_cig_smoking/index.htm. Accessed June 25, 2018.

7: Stanhope KL, Schwarz JM, Keim NL, et al. Consuming fructose-sweetened, not glucose-sweetened, beverages increases visceral adiposity and lipids and decreases insulin sensitivity in overweight/obese humans. *The Journal of Clinical Investigation.* 2009;119(5):1322–1334.

8: Hawkins TR, Gausen OM, Strømman AH. Environmental impacts of hybrid and electric vehicles—a review. *Int J Life Cycle Assess* (2012);17:997.

9: Granovskii M, Dincer I, Rosen MA. Economic and environmental comparison of conventional, hybrid, electric and hydrogen fuel cell vehicles. *Journal of Power Sources.* 2006;159(2):1186–1193.

10: Kaiser J. The dirt on ocean garbage patches. *Science.* 18 Jun 2010;328(5985):1506.

11: Sharma B, Mehta G. Selection of materials for green construction: a review. *IOSR-JMCE.* 2014;11(6) ver III:80–88.

12: https://www.edf.org/attention-drivers-turn-your-idling-engines. Accessed June 25, 2018.

13: Smith-Barbaro P, Hanson D, Reddy BS. Carcinogen binding to various types of dietary fiber. *J Natl Cancer Inst.* 1981 Aug;67(2):495–497.

14: Romero-Franco M, Hernández-Ramírez RU, Calafat AM, Cebrián ME, Needham LL, Teitelbaum S, Wolff MS, López-Carrillo L. Personal care product use and urinary levels of phthalate metabolites in Mexican women. *Environ Int.* 2011 Jul;37(5):867–871.

15: Allmyr M, Adolfsson-Erici M, McLachlan MS, Sandborgh-Englund G. Triclosan in plasma and milk from Swedish nursing mothers and their exposure via personal care products. *Sci Total Environ.* 2006 Dec 15;372(1):87–93.

16: https://davidsuzuki.org/queen-of-green/dirty-dozen-cosmetic-chemicals-avoid. Accessed June 25, 2018.

17: Cai L, Wan D, Yi F, Luan L. Purification, preliminary characterization and hepatoprotective effects of polysaccharides from dandelion root. *Molecules.* 2017 Aug 25;22(9):1409.

18: You Y, Yoo S, Yoon HG, Park J, Lee YH, Kim S, Oh KT, Lee J, Cho HY, Jun W. In vitro and in vivo hepatoprotective effects of the aqueous extract from Taraxacum officinale (dandelion) root against alcohol-induced oxidative stress. *Food Chem Toxicol.* 2010 Jun;48(6):1632–1637.

19: Davaatseren M, Hur HJ, Yang HJ, Hwang JT, Park JH, Kim HJ, Kim MJ, Kwon DY, Sung MJ. Taraxacum official (dandelion) leaf extract alleviates high-fat diet-induced nonalcoholic fatty liver. *Food Chem Toxicol.* 2013 Aug;58:30–36.

20: Federico A, Dallio M, Loguercio C. Silymarin/silybin and chronic liver disease: a marriage of many years. *Molecules.* 2017 Jan 24;22(2):pii: E191.

21: Abenavoli L, Capasso R, Milic N, Capasso F. Milk thistle in liver diseases: past, present, future. *Phytother Res.* 2010 Oct;24(10):1423–1432.

22: Park EJ, Jeon CH, Ko G, Kim J, Sohn DH. Protective effect of curcumin in rat liver injury induced by carbon tetrachloride. *J Pharm Pharmacol.* 2000 Apr;52(4):437–440.

23: Kiso Y, Suzuki Y, Watanabe N, Oshima Y, Hikino H. Antihepatotoxic principles of Curcuma longa rhizomes. *Planta Med.* 1983 Nov;49(3):185–187.

24: Patrick-Iwuanyanwu KC, Wegwu MO, Ayalogu EO. Prevention of CCl4-induced liver damage by ginger, garlic and vitamin E. *Pak J Biol Sci.* 2007 Feb 15;10(4):617–621.

25: Amagase H, Petesch BL, Matsuura H, Kasuga S, Itakura Y. Intake of garlic and its bioactive components. *J Nutr.* 2001 Mar;131(3s):955S–962S.

26: Kreydiyyeh SI, Usta J. Diuretic effect and mechanism of action of parsley. *J Ethnopharmacol.* 2002 Mar;79(3):353–357.

27: Mehmetçik G, Ozdemirler G, Koçak-Toker N, Cevikbaş U, Uysal M. Effect of pretreatment with artichoke extract on carbon tetrachloride-induced liver injury and oxidative stress. *Exp Toxicol Pathol.* 2008 Sep;60(6):475–480.

28: Krajka-Kuźniak V, Paluszczak J, Szaefer H, Baer-Dubowska W. Betanin, a beetroot component, induces nuclear factor erythroid-2-related factor 2-mediated expression of detoxifying/antioxidant enzymes in human liver cell lines. *Br J Nutr.* 2013 Dec;110(12):2138–2149.

29: Váli L, Stefanovits-Bányai E, Szentmihályi K, Fébel H, Sárdi E, Lugasi A, Kocsis I, Blázovics A. Liver-protecting effects of table beet (Beta vulgaris var. rubra) during ischemia-reperfusion. *Nutrition.* 2007 Feb;23(2):172–178.

30: Kim BY, Cui ZG, Lee SR, Kim SJ, Kang HK, Lee YK, Park DB. Effects of Asparagus officinalis extracts on liver cell toxicity and ethanol metabolism. *J Food Sci.* 2009 Sep;74(7):H204–208.

31: Zhu X, Zhang W, Zhao J, Wang J, Qu W. Hypolipidaemic and hepatoprotective effects of ethanolic and aqueous extracts from Asparagus officinalis L. by-products in mice fed a high-fat diet. *J Sci Food Agric.* 2010 May;90(7):1129–1135.

32: Kim MJ, Hwang JH, Ko HJ, Na HB, Kim JH. Lemon detox diet reduced body fat, insulin resistance, and serum hs-CRP level without hematological changes in overweight Korean women. *Nutr Res.* 2015 May;35(5):409–420.

33: Vanuytsel T, van Wanrooy S, Vanheel H, Vanormelingen C, Verschueren S, Houben E, Salim Rasoel S, Tóth J, Holvoet L, Farré R, Van Oudenhove L, Boeckxstaens G, Verbeke K, Tack J. Psychological stress and corticotropin-releasing hormone increase intestinal permeability in humans by a mast cell-dependent mechanism. *Gut.* 2014 Aug;63(8):1293–1299.

Cancer

1: Soto AM, Sonnenschein C. Environmental causes of cancer: endocrine disruptors as carcinogens. *Nat Rev Endocrinol.* 2010 Jul;6(7):363–370.

2: Langie SA, Koppen G, Desaulniers D, Al-Mulla F, Al-Temaimi R, Amedei A, Azqueta A, Bisson WH, Brown DG, Brunborg G, Charles AK, Chen T, Colacci A, Darroudi F, Forte S, Gonzalez L, Hamid RA, Knudsen LE, Leyns L, Lopez de Cerain Salsamendi A, Memeo L, Mondello C, Mothersill C, Olsen AK, Pavanello S, Raju J, Rojas E, Roy R, Ryan EP, Ostrosky-Wegman P, Salem HK, Scovassi AI, Singh N, Vaccari M, Van Schooten FJ, Valverde M, Woodrick J, Zhang L, van Larebeke N, Kirsch-Volders M, Collins AR. Causes of genome instability: the effect of low dose chemical exposures in modern society. *Carcinogenesis.* 2015 Jun;36 Suppl1:S61–88.

3: Seyfried TN. Cancer as a mitochondrial metabolic disease. *Frontiers in Cell and Developmental Biology.* 2015;3:43.

4: Christofferson T. *Tripping over the Truth: The Metabolic Theory of Cancer.* CreateSpace. 2014.

5: Cisneros L, Bussey KJ, Orr AJ, Miočević M, Lineweaver CH, Davies P. Ancient genes establish stress-induced mutation as a hallmark of cancer. Galli A, ed. *PLoS ONE.* 2017;12(4):e0176258.

6: Lineweaver CH, Davies PCW, Vincent MD. Targeting cancer's weaknesses (not its strengths): therapeutic strategies suggested by the atavistic model. *BioEssays: News and Reviews in Molecular, Cellular and Developmental Biology.* 2014;36(9):827–835.

7: Moen I, Stuhr LEB. Hyperbaric oxygen therapy and cancer—a review. *Targeted Oncology.* 2012;7(4):233–242.

8: http://nutritiondata.self.com. Searched under tools; nutrient search tool; foods highest in iron. Accessed May 12, 2018.

9: Garland CF, Gorham ED, Mohr SB, Garland FC. Vitamin D for cancer prevention: global perspective. *Ann Epidemiol.* 2009 Jul;19(7):468–483.

10: Palacios C, Gonzalez L. Is vitamin D deficiency a major global public health problem? *The Journal of Steroid Biochemistry and Molecular Biology.* 2014;144PA:138–145.

11: Nair R, Maseeh A. Vitamin D: the "sunshine" vitamin. *Journal of Pharmacology & Pharmacotherapeutics.* 2012;3(2):118–126.

12: https://www.vitamindcouncil.org/about-vitamin-d/how-do-i-get-the-vitamin-d-my-body-needs. Accessed May 24, 2018.

13: Gallagher RP, Hill GB, Bajdik CD, Fincham S, Coldman AJ, McLean DI, Threlfall WJ. Sunlight exposure, pigmentary factors, and risk of nonmelanocytic skin cancer. I. Basal cell carcinoma. *Arch Dermatol.* 1995 Feb;131(2):157–163.

14: Butt ST, Christensen T. Toxicity and phototoxicity of chemical sun filters. *Radiation Protection Dosimetry.* 2000 Sept;91(1-3):283–286.

15: http://nutritiondata.self.com. Searched under tools; nutrient search tool; foods highest in Vitamin D. Accessed May 10, 2018.

16: Borek C. Antioxidant health effects of aged garlic extract. *J Nutr.* 2001 Mar;131(3s):1010S-1015S.

17: Amagase H, Petesch BL, Matsuura H, Kasuga S, Itakura Y. Intake of garlic and its bioactive components. *J Nutr.* 2001 Mar;131(3s):955S–962S.

18: Ni CX, Gong H, Liu Y, Qi Y, Jiang CL, Zhang JP. Green tea consumption and the risk of liver cancer: a meta-analysis. *Nutr Cancer.* 2017 Feb-Mar;69(2):211–220.

19: Krajka-Kuźniak V, Paluszczak J, Szaefer H, Baer-Dubowska W. Betanin, a beetroot component, induces nuclear factor erythroid-2-related factor 2-mediated expression of detoxifying/antioxidant enzymes in human liver cell lines. *Br J Nutr.* 2013 Dec;110(12):2138–2149.

20: Chattopadhyay I, Biswas K, Bandyopadhyay U, Banerjee R. Turmeric and curcumin: biological actions and medicinal applications. *Current Science.* 2004;87(1):44–53.

21: Park W, Amin AR, Chen ZG, Shin DM. New perspectives of curcumin in cancer prevention. *Cancer Prev Res* (Phila). 2013 May;6(5):387–400.

22: Higdon JV, Delage B, Williams DE, Dashwood RH. Cruciferous vegetables and human cancer risk: epidemiologic evidence and mechanistic basis. *Pharmacological Research: The Official Journal of the Italian Pharmacological Society.* 2007;55(3):224–236.

23: Murillo G, Mehta RG. Cruciferous vegetables and cancer prevention. *Nutr Cancer.* 2001;41(1-2):17–28.

24: Sun W, Wang W, Kim J, Keng P, Yang S, Zhang H, Liu C, Okunieff P, Zhang L. Anti-cancer effect of resveratrol is associated with induction of apoptosis via a mitochondrial pathway alignment. *Adv Exp Med Biol.* 2008;614:179–186.

25: Jang M, Cai L, Udeani GO, Slowing KV, Thomas CF, Beecher CW, Fong HH, Farnsworth NR, Kinghorn AD, Mehta RG, Moon RC, Pezzuto JM. Cancer chemopreventive activity of resveratrol, a natural product derived from grapes. *Science.* 1997 Jan 10;275(5297):218–220.

26: Anderson RM, Shanmuganayagam D, Weindruch R. Caloric restriction and aging: studies in mice and monkeys. *Toxicol Pathol.* 2009 Jan;37(1):47–51.

27: Heilbronn LK, de Jonge L, Frisard MI, DeLany JP, Larson-Meyer DE, Rood J, Nguyen T, Martin CK, Volaufova J, Most MM, Greenway FL, Smith SR, Deutsch WA, Williamson DA, Ravussin E; Pennington CALERIE Team. Effect of 6-month calorie restriction on biomarkers of longevity, metabolic adaptation, and oxidative stress in overweight individuals: a randomized controlled trial. *JAMA.* 2006 Apr 5;295(13):1539–1548. Erratum in: *JAMA.* 2006 Jun 7;295(21):2482.

28: Cheng CW, Adams GB, Perin L, Wei M, Zhou X, Lam BS, Da Sacco S, Mirisola M, Quinn DI, Dorff TB, Kopchick JJ, Longo VD. Prolonged fasting reduces IGF-1/PKA to promote hematopoietic-stem-cell-based regeneration and reverse immunosuppression. *Cell Stem Cell.* 2014 Jun 5;14(6):810–823.

29: Safdie FM, Dorff T, Quinn D, Fontana L, Wei M, Lee C, Cohen P, Longo VD. Fasting and cancer treatment in humans: a case series report. *Aging (Albany NY)*. 2009 Dec 31;1(12):988–1007.

Weight Loss

1: McGee DL; Diverse Populations Collaboration. Body mass index and mortality: a meta-analysis based on person-level data from twenty-six observational studies. *Ann Epidemiol*. 2005 Feb;15(2):87–97.

2: Pischon T, Sharma AM. Use of beta-blockers in obesity hypertension: potential role of weight gain. *Obes Rev*. 2001 Nov;2(4):275–280.

3: Fava M. Weight gain and antidepressants. *J Clin Psychiatry*. 2000;61 Suppl 11:37–41.

4: Soeters MR, Lammers NM, Dubbelhuis PF, Ackermans M, Jonkers-Schuitema CF, Fliers E, Sauerwein HP, Aerts JM, Serlie MJ. Intermittent fasting does not affect whole-body glucose, lipid, or protein metabolism. *Am J Clin Nutr*. 2009 Nov;90(5):1244–1251.

5: https://www.motherjones.com/environment/2015/03/against-meals-breakfast-lunch-dinner. Accessed May 17, 2018.

6: Azevedo FR, Ikeoka D, Caramelli B. Effects of intermittent fasting on metabolism in men. *Rev Assoc Med Bras* (1992). 2013 Mar-Apr;59(2):167–173.

7: Klempel MC, Kroeger CM, Bhutani S, Trepanowski JF, Varady KA. Intermittent fasting combined with calorie restriction is effective for weight loss and cardio-protection in obese women. *Nutr J*. 2012 Nov 21;11:98.

8: White AM, Johnston CS. Vinegar ingestion at bedtime moderates waking glucose concentrations in adults with well-controlled type 2 diabetes. *Diabetes Care*. 2007 Nov;30(11):2814–2815.

9: Johnston CS, Steplewska I, Long CA, Harris LN, Ryals RH. Examination of the antiglycemic properties of vinegar in healthy adults. *Ann Nutr Metab*. 2010;56(1):74–79.

10: Budak NH, Aykin E, Seydim AC, Greene AK, Guzel-Seydim ZB. Functional properties of vinegar. *J Food Sci*. 2014 May;79(5):R757–764.

11: Kirkham S, Akilen R, Sharma S, Tsiami A. The potential of cinnamon to reduce blood glucose levels in patients with type 2 diabetes and insulin resistance. *Diabetes Obes Metab*. 2009 Dec;11(12):1100–1113.

12: Davis C, Bryan J, Hodgson J, Murphy K. Definition of the Mediterranean diet; a literature review. *Nutrients*. 2015 Nov 5;7(11):9139–9153.

13: Keene DL. A systematic review of the use of the ketogenic diet in childhood epilepsy. *Pediatr Neurol*. 2006 Jul;35(1):1–5.

14: Gasior M, Rogawski MA, Hartman AL. Neuroprotective and disease-modifying effects of the ketogenic diet. *Behavioural Pharmacology*. 2006;17(5-6):431–439.

15: Brehm BJ, Seeley RJ, Daniels SR, D'Alessio DA. A randomized trial comparing a very low carbohydrate diet and a calorie-restricted low fat diet on body weight and cardiovascular risk factors in healthy women. *J Clin Endocrinol Metab*. 2003 Apr;88(4):1617–1623.

16: Millichap JG, Jones JD. Acid-base, electrolyte, and amino-acid metabolism in children with petit mai. Etiologic significance and modification by anticonvulsant drugs and the ketogenic diet. *Epilepsia*.1964;5:239–255.

Healthy Pregnancy

1: Kort JD, Winget C, Kim SH, Lathi RB. A retrospective cohort study to evaluate the impact of meaningful weight loss on fertility outcomes in an overweight population with infertility. *Fertil Steril*. 2014 May;101(5):1400–1403.

2: Clark AM, Thornley B, Tomlinson L, Galletley C, Norman RJ. Weight loss in obese infertile women results in improvement in reproductive outcome for all forms of fertility treatment. *Hum Reprod.* 1998 Jun;13(6):1502–1505.

3: Warren MP, Perlroth NE. The effects of intense exercise on the female reproductive system. *J Endocrinol.* 2001 Jul;170(1):3–11.

4: Sanders KA, Bruce NW. A prospective study of psychosocial stress and fertility in women. *Hum Reprod.* 1997 Oct;12(10):2324–2329.

5: Gollenberg AL, Liu F, Brazil C, Drobnis EZ, Guzick D, Overstreet JW, Redmon JB, Sparks A, Wang C, Swan SH. Semen quality in fertile men in relation to psychosocial stress. *Fertil Steril.* 2010 Mar 1;93(4):1104–1111.

6: Windham GC, Hopkins B, Fenster L, Swan SH. Prenatal active or passive tobacco smoke exposure and the risk of preterm delivery or low birth weight. *Epidemiology.* 2000 Jul;11(4):427–433.

7: Bhuvaneswar CG, Chang G, Epstein LA, Stern TA. Alcohol use during pregnancy: prevalence and impact. *Primary Care Companion to The Journal of Clinical Psychiatry.* 2007;9(6):455–460.

8: Chen LW, Wu Y, Neelakantan N, Chong MF, Pan A, van Dam RM. Maternal caffeine intake during pregnancy is associated with risk of low birth weight: a systematic review and dose-response meta-analysis. *BMC Med.* 2014 Sep 19;12:174.

9: Chaudhry SA, Gad N, Koren G. Toxoplasmosis and pregnancy. *Canadian Family Physician.* 2014;60(4):334–336.

10: https://www.foodsafety.gov/risk/pregnant. Accessed June 26, 2018.

11: Maciocia G. *The Foundations of Chinese Medicine: A Comprehensive Text for Acupuncturist and Herbalist.* 2nd ed. 2005.

12: Haddow JE, Palomaki GE, Allan WC, Williams JR, Knight GJ, Gagnon J, O'Heir CE, Mitchell ML, Hermos RJ, Waisbren SE, Faix JD, Klein RZ. Maternal thyroid deficiency during pregnancy and subsequent neuropsychological development of the child. *N Engl J Med.* 1999 Aug 19;341(8):549–555.

13: Salvesen KA, Mørkved S. Randomised controlled trial of pelvic floor muscle training during pregnancy. *BMJ.* 2004 Aug 14;329(7462):378–380.

14: Harvey MA. Pelvic floor exercises during and after pregnancy: a systematic review of their role in preventing pelvic floor dysfunction. *J Obstet Gynaecol Can.* 2003 Jun;25(6):487–498.

15: Holst L, Haavik S, Nordeng H. Raspberry leaf—should it be recommended to pregnant women? *Complement Ther Clin Pract.* 2009 Nov;15(4):204–208.

16: http://www.upmc.com/patients-visitors/education/pregnancy/Pages/caring-for -yourself-after-you-have-your-baby.aspx. Accessed June 26, 2018.

17: Ramler D, Roberts J. A comparison of cold and warm sitz baths for relief of postpartum perineal pain. *J Obstet Gynecol Neonatal Nurs.* 1986 Nov-Dec;15(6):471–474.

18: https://www.emedicinehealth.com/postpartum_perineal_care/article_ em.htm#perineum_care_at_home. Accessed June 26, 2018.

19: https://my.clevelandclinic.org/health/articles/9682-pregnancy-physical-changes-after-delivery. Accessed June 26, 2018.

20: Ibid.

21: https://www.womenshealth.gov/pregnancy/childbirth-and-beyond/recovering-birth. Accessed June 26, 2018.

22: https://my.clevelandclinic.org/health/articles/9682-pregnancy-physical-changes-after-delivery. Accessed June 26, 2018.

23: https://kidshealth.org/en/parents/pregnancy.html. Accessed June 26, 2018.

24: https://my.clevelandclinic.org/health/articles/9682-pregnancy-physical-changes-after-delivery. Accessed June 26, 2018.

25: https://kidshealth.org/en/parents/pregnancy.html. Accessed June 26, 2018.

Healthy Children

1: http://www.who.int/maternal_child_adolescent/topics/newborn/nutrition/breastfeeding/en. Accessed June 28, 2018.

2: https://kidshealth.org/en/parents/breast-bottle-feeding.html. Accessed June 28, 2018.

3: http://www.who.int/maternal_child_adolescent/topics/newborn/nutrition/breastfeeding/en. Accessed June 28, 2018.

4: https://kidshealth.org/en/parents/breast-bottle-feeding.html. Accessed June 28, 2018.

5: https://www.aap.org/en-us/advocacy-and-policy/aap-health-initiatives/Breastfeeding/Pages/Benefits-of-Breastfeeding.aspx. Accessed June 28, 2018.

6: https://www.mayoclinic.org/diseases-conditions/peanut-allergy/symptoms-causes/syc-20376175. Accessed June 29, 2018.

7: Fleischer DM, Sicherer S, Greenhawt M, Campbell D, Chan E, Muraro A, Halken S, Katz Y, Ebisawa M, Eichenfield L, Sampson H, Lack G, Du Toit G, Roberts G, Bahnson H, Feeney M, Hourihane J, Spergel J, Young M, As'aad A, Allen K, Prescott S, Kapur S, Saito H, Agache I, Akdis CA, Arshad H, Beyer K, Dubois A, Eigenmann P, Fernandez-Rivas M, Grimshaw K, Hoffman-Sommergruber K, Host A, Lau S, O'Mahony L, Mills C, Papadopoulos N, Venter C, Agmon-Levin N, Kessel A, Antaya R, Drolet B, Rosenwasser L. Consensus communication on early peanut introduction and the prevention of peanut allergy in high-risk infants. *Ann Allergy Asthma Immunol.* 2015 Aug;115(2):87–90.

8: Du Toit G, Katz Y, Sasieni P, Mesher D, Maleki SJ, Fisher HR, Fox AT, Turcanu V, Amir T, Zadik-Mnuhin G, Cohen A, Livne I, Lack G. Early consumption of peanuts in infancy is associated with a low prevalence of peanut allergy. *J Allergy Clin Immunol.* 2008 Nov;122(5):984–991.

9: https://www.mayoclinic.org/diseases-conditions/peanut-allergy/symptoms-causes/syc-20376175. Accessed June 29, 2018.

10: Alhassan M, Ansong D, Ampomah AO, Albritton TJ. Junior high school students' use of their afterschool hours in Ghana: the role of household assets. *Child & Youth Services.* 2017;38(3):231–251.

11: Michaud I, Chaput JP, O'Loughlin J, Tremblay A, Mathieu ME. Long duration of stressful homework as a potential obesogenic factor in children: a QUALITY study. *Obesity (Silver Spring).* 2015 Apr;23(4):815–822.

12: https://www.southuniversity.edu/whoweare/newsroom/blog/the-advantages-of-family-time-113366. Accessed June 29, 2018.

13: https://greatergood.berkeley.edu/images/uploads/Parent_Tips_-_Raising_Caring_Children.pdf. Accessed June 29, 2018.

14: https://centerforparentingeducation.org/library-of-articles/healthy-communication/the-skill-of-listening. Accessed May 22, 2018.

15: https://greatergood.berkeley.edu/images/uploads/Parent_Tips_-_Raising_Caring_Children.pdf. Accessed June 29, 2018.

16: https://centerforparentingeducation.org/library-of-articles/healthy-communication/the-skill-of-listening. Accessed May 22, 2018.

17: http://raisingchildren.net.au/articles/praise_and_encouragement.html. Accessed May 23, 2018.

18: Mueller CM, Dweck CS. Praise for intelligence can undermine children's motivation and performance. *J Pers Soc Psychol.* 1998 Jul;75(1):33–52.

19: http://raisingchildren.net.au/articles/discipline_teenagers.html. Accessed June 29, 2018.

20: https://www.parentingforbrain.com/children-hugging. Accessed May 23, 2018.

21: Thoma MV, La Marca R, Brönnimann R, Finkel L, Ehlert U, Nater UM. The effect of music on the human stress response. Newton RL, ed. *PLoS ONE*. 2013;8(8):e70156.

22: https://med.stanford.edu/news/all-news/2007/07/music-moves-brain-to-pay-attention-stanford-study-finds.html. Accessed June 29, 2018.

23: https://www.unr.edu/counseling/virtual-relaxation-room/releasing-stress-through-the-power-of-music. Accessed June 29, 2018.

24: Črnčec R, Wilson SJ, Prior M. The cognitive and academic benefits of music to children: facts and fiction. *Educational Psychology*. 2006;26:4,579–594.

25: Hillman CH, Castelli DM, Buck SM. Aerobic fitness and neurocognitive function in healthy preadolescent children. *Med Sci Sports Exerc*. 2005 Nov;37(11):1967–1174.

26: Guidelines for School and Community Programs to Promote Lifelong Physical Activity Among Young People, March 07, 1997 / 46(RR-6);1-36. https://www.cdc.gov/mmwr/preview/mmwrhtml/00046823.htm. Accessed May 23, 2018.

27: Callahan GN. Eating dirt. *Emerging Infectious Diseases*. 2003;9(8):1016–1021.

28: Smaldone A, Honig JC, Byrne MW. Sleepless in America: inadequate sleep and relationships to health and well-being of our nation's children. *Pediatrics*. 2007 Feb;119 Suppl 1:S29–37.

29: https://sleepfoundation.org/press-release/national-sleep-foundation-recommends-new-sleep-times. Accessed May 24, 2018.

30: https://kidshealth.org/en/parents/naps.html. Accessed June 29, 2018.

Aging

1: Mäkelä P. Alcohol-related mortality by age and sex and its impact on life expectancy: estimates based on the Finnish death register. *European Journal of Public Health*. 1998 March 1;8(1):43–51.

2: Ferrucci L, Izmirlian G, Leveille S, Phillips CL, Corti MC, Brock DB, Guralnik JM. Smoking, physical activity, and active life expectancy. *Am J Epidemiol*. 1999 Apr 1;149(7):645-653.

3: Shigenaga MK, Hagen TM, Ames BN. Oxidative damage and mitochondrial decay in aging. *Proc Natl Acad Sci U S A*. 1994 Nov 8;91(23):10771-10778.

4: https://www.ars.usda.gov/news-events/news/research-news/1999/high-orac-foods-may-slow-aging. Accessed May 26, 2018.

5: Chen J, Li Y, Zhu Q, Li T, Lu H, Wei N, Huang Y, Shi R, Ma X, Wang X, Sheng J. Anti-skin-aging effect of epigallocatechin gallate by regulating epidermal growth factor receptor pathway on aging mouse model induced by d-Galactose. *Mech Ageing Dev*. 2017 Jun;164:1–7.

6: Li YH, Wu Y, Wei HC, Xu YY, Jia LL, Chen J, Yang XS, Dong GH, Gao XH, Chen HD. Protective effects of green tea extracts on photoaging and photoimmunosuppression. *Skin Res Technol*. 2009 Aug;15(3):338–345.

7: Bagchi D, Sen CK, Bagchi M, Atalay M. Anti-angiogenic, antioxidant, and anti-carcinogenic properties of a novel anthocyanin-rich berry extract formula. *Biochemistry (Mosc)*. 2004 Jan;69(1):75–80.

8: Zafra-Stone S, Yasmin T, Bagchi M, Chatterjee A, Vinson JA, Bagchi D. Berry anthocyanins as novel antioxidants in human health and disease prevention. *Mol Nutr Food Res*. 2007 Jun;51(6):675–683.

9: Verhagen H, Poulsen HE, Loft S, van Poppel G, Willems MI, van Bladeren PJ. Reduction of oxidative DNA-damage in humans by brussels sprouts. *Carcinogenesis*. 1995 Apr;16(4):969–970.

10: Shoba G, Joy D, Joseph T, Majeed M, Rajendran R, Srinivas PS. Influence of piperine on the pharmacokinetics of curcumin in animals and human volunteers. *Planta Med*. 1998;64(4):353–356.

11: Srivastava S. The mitochondrial basis of aging and age-related disorders. *Genes*. 2017;8(12):398.

12: Muoio DM, Newgard CB. Obesity-related derangements in metabolic regulation. *Annu Rev Biochem*. 2006;75:367–401.

13: Cioffi F, Senese R, Lasala P, Ziello A, Mazzoli A, Crescenzo R, Liverini G, Lanni A, Goglia F, Iossa S. Fructose-rich diet affects mitochondrial DNA damage and repair in rats. *Nutrients*. 2017 Mar 24;9(4).

14: Donges CE, Burd NA, Duffield R, Smith GC, West DW, Short MJ, Mackenzie R, Plank LD, Shepherd PR, Phillips SM, Edge JA. Concurrent resistance and aerobic exercise stimulates both myofibrillar and mitochondrial protein synthesis in sedentary middle-aged men. *J Appl Physiol* (1985). 2012 Jun;112(12):1992–2001.

15: Fetterman JL, Sammy MJ, Ballinger SW. Mitochondrial toxicity of tobacco smoke and air pollution. *Toxicology*. 2017 Nov 1;391:18–33.

About the Author

Dr. Behzad Azargoshasb, ND, is a naturopathic doctor practicing in Ontario, Canada; an avid writer featured in HubPages; and an author. He spends his days helping people from all walks of life improve their health through natural, noninvasive methods. He is loved by his patients and followers for bringing hope and health back into their lives. His clinical focus is on digestive health, autoimmune conditions, and metabolic disorders. His passion is to educate and motivate his patients into health-promoting lifestyles. Good health is your God-given right, and Dr. Behzad wants to put the power back into your hands by empowering you with credible and useful knowledge through His works.

Scan to visit

therulesofhealth.com